BLESSED ARE THE CAREGIVERS

PRACTICAL ADVICE AND ECOURAGEMENT

FOR THOSE PROVIDING CARE TO OTHERS

DANNY CAIN
AND
BOB RUSSELL

BLESSED ARE THE CAREGIVERS

Library of Congress Catalog No.: 95-069557

ISBN: 0-9646630-0-7

95   1

Blessed Are The Caregivers

A Practical and Spiritual Guide for Caregivers of Alzheimer's Patients

ISOLATION 1

ANGER
    (BEHAVIOR CHANGES) 3

POWERLESSNESS 5

SELF-DOUBT 7

LONELINESS 9

WANDERING 11

GUILT 13

EMBARRASSMENT
    (UNDRESSING) 15

INCONTINENCE 17

ABANDONMENT
    (FAMILY) 19

DISTRESS
    (NEW RESPONSIBILITIES) 21

SUFFERING
    (INJURIES) 23

LETTING GO 25

FIDGETING 27

FAITH
    (TRUST) 29

FEAR
    (HEREDITARY) 31

COMPANIONSHIP 35

DISTANCE
    (PERSONAL) 37

CLINGING 39

HOARDING 41

COMMUNICATION 45

GORGING 47

RIGIDITY 49

INFANTILIZATION 51

SUBTLE CHANGES 53

CUING
    (PROMPTING) 55

ECHOLALIA
    (SPEECH) 57

SELF - PITY 59

LOVE 61

MISUNDERSTANDING 63

AWARENESS 65

RUSHING 67

CONTROL 69

SHAME 71

ACHIEVEMENT 73

ATTITUDE 75

REMINISCING
    (RECALL) 77

BATHING 79

DRIVING 81

COPING 83

MOURNING 85

PARANOIA 87

TRUST 89

FALLS 91

SWALLOWING
    (NOURISHMENT) 93

AGGRESSION 95

HALLUCINATION 97

INTIMACY 99

PLACEMENT 101

FABRICATION 103

TREMORS 105

AGNOSIA
    (RECOGNITION) 107

ALZHEIMER'S DISEASE OVERVIEW 109

Preface

This book is dedicated to all of the caregivers who give endlessly of their love, time and patience caring for individuals with Alzheimer's disease. I want to especially thank those families that have been members of my support group these past twelve years. I hope and pray that someday soon we'll find the cause and cure to this devastating illness.

The real joy of writing this book was the satisfaction that I've received from being able to give back but a small portion of what God has provided for me all of these years.

A special note of thanks and gratitude to my wife Jo-e, whose on-going support and love have meant so much to me. Her editing and commentary reviews allowed me to fine tune the language and make it more user friendly. I would not have taken on the challenge of writing *Blessed are the Caregivers* had it not been for the help of my co-author, Bob Russell. He has truly been an inspiration to me and my family. The fact that our paths crossed wasn't by coincidence, but rather, as Bob often says, a God incidence. How true!

Introduction

The idea of writing *Blessed are the Caregivers* started some twelve years ago when I began leading my first support group for caregivers of Alzheimer's patients. Little did I know that this idea wouldn't take on meaning until the fall of 1993. While attending Southeast Christian Church I was introduced to the pastor and my co-author Bob Russell. His practical biblical-based approach to life helped me grow in my own personal walk. I know that the Lord had his hand in this encounter.

I had sketched out a format for a book that I felt would serve the spiritual needs of caregivers. My previous experience working with support groups had identified certain individuals who impressed me. These group members seemed to have a strong conviction and spiritual commitment that was reflected in their walk as caregivers. More amazing was the way they handled adversity and the special burdens that were placed upon them on a day-to-day basis. These individuals should truly be blessed for their efforts, I thought. So came the name, *Blessed are the Caregivers.*

But what did I know about writing a practical guide addressing the spiritual needs of caregivers? My experience was focused towards the clinical side of this disease. I could easily discuss the symptoms and stages of this illness but I felt that I really needed assistance with addressing issues of caregiver faith. Several months had passed and I realized how fortunate my family had been in attending this church. Bob's sermons were so meaningful and to the point. After several preliminary meetings we agreed to write this book together.

Blessed are the Caregivers is a hands-on practical approach which depicts real life situations that caregivers can use in providing their loved ones' care. The most effective caregiver who ever lived was Jesus Christ. He touched people society considered untouchable. He took time for the people society ignored. He loved the unlovely and brought healing and compassion to the terminally ill.

Jesus encouraged us to love as He loved. He said, "As I have loved you, so you ought also to love one another." It's most appropriate, therefore, that a book intended to encourage caregivers should include inspirational thoughts from the primary source of love and compassion — Jesus Christ. "The same as you do it to the least of these you did for me" (Matthew 25:40).

Both authors have attempted to provide the reader with a strong sense of association and relevance to the issues confronting caregivers. Bob's story-like messages and scriptural references serve to provide the caregiver with the necessary tools to enhance one's faith and spiritual belief. The daily tasks and challenges of caregiving lend themselves to further self-study and this book provides the reader with an excellent roadmap to navigate the difficult and sometimes unrewarding duties of a caregiver.

We both hope and pray that your walk as a caregiver will be blessed with a strong sense of faith and commitment and that your life will grow closer to the Lord as a result of this experience. God bless.

ISOLATION

*S*ince my husband has been diagnosed as having Alzheimer's Disease, I feel lonely and abandoned by my friends. They no longer call me as they used to, and I am uneasy discussing Bill's peculiar behavior. I stay busy and so over-worked that I no longer have the time to get out and be a part of their circles.

Practical Suggestions

Isolation refers to the separation of the person from social contact or interaction. Emotional and psychological withdrawal may occur if you fear making contact with other people due to feeling embarrassed. Symptoms include poor self-image, feeling helpless or powerless, having difficulty with establishing goals or making decisions and feeling confined and trapped.

Schedule some time for yourself and explore alternative social functions that allow you to meet and interact with others. Social isolation and deprivation can have a significant effect on the caregiver's well-being. As caregivers become distanced from their support networks, a sense of feeling overwhelmed by the responsibility of caregiving may add to their stress.

A common intervention for isolation is to engage in opportunities that allow you to make choices and to establish realistic goals. Making decisions and being actively engaged in social activities serve to greatly reduce the sense of isolation and loneliness. Link up with a family support group and seek professional guidance if necessary.

Devotional

Jesus also felt alone at times. But He deliberately gathered close friends around Him in times of need. He took with Him into the Garden of Gethsemane Peter, James and John and asked them to join Him in prayer. He was disappointed that they did not fully understand His hurts (they fell asleep!), but He needed them and welcomed their friendship.

Force yourself to be with others even when you don't feel like it. One psychologist said, "If you act the way you wish you felt, you'll eventually feel the way you act." Tell your friends how you're feeling when the appropriate time arises. Give them a chance to lift you up. They may not understand completely but their companionship can help you.

Remember also that Jesus is "a friend who sticks closer than a brother." He understands completely and he has promised, "I will never forsake you."

The champion horse in the Calgary Stampede pulled a little over 9,000 pounds. The horse that came in second pulled just under 9,000 pounds. The horse pull concluded with a demonstration of the horses pulling in tandem. Bets were taken on how much the horses could do together. The crowd was amazed when the two horses pulled 27,000 pounds! There is special strength in pulling together. "Carry each other's burdens and in this way you will fulfill the law of Christ" (Galatians 6:2).

ANGER
(BEHAVIOR CHANGES)

T oday my anger with Mary became more than I could handle. She kept asking me the same question over and over again after I had already answered her. Sometimes I wonder if she is deliberately doing this to upset me. I find myself arguing with her over trivial things that shouldn't bother me. I must continue to remind myself that her behavior is the result of the disease and that her actions are not intentional.

Practical Suggestions

Anger is often expressed through a strong feeling of displeasure or rage. Often caregivers will attempt to rationalize their concerns with their loved one, not realizing that the individual is unable to comprehend what is going on or to control his or her behavior. When this situation presents itself to you, remove yourself from the situation and focus your efforts on something else. If the caregiver has difficulty attempting to change the subject, the use of distraction or diversion may often help by redirecting the individual's attention. Keep in mind that the individual is unable to fully comprehend what is being asked due to a disease.

The caregiver should maintain a calm, positive attitude. When possible, verbally address your feelings of anger and frustration to someone who is supportive and understanding of your concerns. Rechannel hostile feelings into positive activities such as exercise or working on a project. Remember, anger that you allow to be "bottled up" inside of you may cause adverse effects such as high blood pressure and other health problems.

Support groups are often a good resource for caregivers as they provide a high level of commonality and a strong sense of "having been there before." Make time to share your personal feelings and to ventilate caregiving issues.

Devotional

Circumstances beyond your control can be exasperating at times. You can be thankful that the Bible never says "Don't be angry." Instead we are commanded, "In your anger do not sin. Do not let the sun go down while you are angry. Do not give the devil a foothold" (Ephesians 4:26).

Though it is not a sin to be angry, God does warn us to be slow to anger, "for man's anger does not bring about the righteous life that God desires" (James 1:20). Because it is a dangerous emotion, we should pray that God will help us overcome our anger and then work to properly release it.

Ventilating your anger is not the solution. To act out your anger only serves as a temporary relief. Later, when you face the results of your behavior, you may discover that your actions only exacerbated the problems. Instead of taking out your anger on the loved one who frustrates you, express it to God, who understands. Then release your anger by showing kindness. Try doing something special for your dependent again. Whether or not your action is appreciated, it is still the best way to get rid of bitterness.

A sheep farmer was disturbed because his neighbor's dog was killing his lambs. Though he had confronted his neighbor, the dog was never controlled. But instead of suing the neighbor or getting into a bitter argument, he gave a little lamb to his neighbor's children. The dog was soon tied up. "Don't be overcome with evil, but overcome evil with good" (Romans 12:21).

"Get rid of all bitterness, rage and anger, brawling and slander, along with every form of malice. Be kind and compassionate to one another, forgiving one another just as in Christ, God forgave you" (Ephesians 4:32).

POWERLESSNESS

They say that anxiety is the fear of the unknown. I really can relate to that. Since my wife was first diagnosed with Alzheimer's Disease, our lives have been filled with a lot of unforeseen setbacks. How long will this disease go on before it renders her unable to recognize our children or even me? Some days, she seems better than others only to then fall back a step or two. It's an emotional roller coaster. I don't know what to expect next.

Practical Suggestions

Caregiving often involves a personal awareness and feeling of being powerless. One may feel unable to change an impending and almost inevitable event or behavior. Have you ever heard the expression, "Where there is hope, there is life?" This expression is especially true for caregivers of Alzheimer's patients.

Often, there doesn't seem to be a lot of hope. Daily activities become nearly impossible to complete. The future doesn't give much hope of getting better as your responsibilities increase. Yet, through it all, you somehow miraculously seem to do the impossible.

Caregivers can accomplish many things when they set their minds to it. Remember to keep your plan of attack simple and straightforward. Break down your action plans into small achievable steps. Be careful not to set yourself up for disappointment or failure. Your goals should not be unrealistic or difficult to obtain. Success in small accomplishments builds one's self-esteem.

Devotional

One of the most important and difficult lessons God wants

5

us to learn about life is that we are not in control — He is. "Trust in the Lord with all your heart and lean not on your own understanding . . ." (Proverbs 3:5).

In our pride we like to think we can control our own destiny. Man boasts, "I'm the captain of my soul, I'm the master of my fate." But in reality, nothing in this world is certain. We have very little control of our future. Wealth, relationships, jobs and health may seem secure at the present time, but they can be taken from us in a moment.

James wrote, "Now listen, you who say, 'Today or tomorrow we will go to this or that city, spend a year there, carry on business and make money.' Why, you do not even know what will happen tomorrow. What is your life? You are a mist that appears for a little while and then vanishes. Instead, you ought to say, 'If it is the Lord's will, we will live and do this or that.' As it is, you boast and brag. All such boasting is evil" (James 4:13-16).

Only when we put our trust completely in God will we experience true security and stability. "It wasn't until God was all I had that I realized He was all I needed," said one saint.

We are often like the elderly woman who was terrified of flying. After her first trip on a commercial jet, she admitted that it wasn't as bad as she thought it would be, but added, "I never did relax enough to put my whole weight down!"

Though the future seems uncertain, put your trust in the Lord today. He is the only one who is in complete control. Someone said, "I don't know what the future holds, but I know who holds the future."

"God alone is my rock and my salvation; He is my fortress, I will never be shaken" (Psalm 62:2).

SELF-DOUBT

E*ach day the task of caring for my wife becomes more difficult and testing. I ask myself time after time, "How long can I continue to care for her many needs?" My ability to continue with this responsibility places an enormous weight put on my shoulders. Lord, give me the strength to do my best for the one I love dearly.*

Practical Suggestions

A feeling of uncertainty may play on the mind of the caregiver. This feeling may be difficult to overcome and may leave the individual preoccupied or obsessed with his or her caregiving abilities. Positive reinforcement and success in one's areas of perceived caregiving weaknesses can give way to confidence and positive self-esteem.

Network with family and friends and get involved in a local support group. Sharing your accomplishments with other caregivers allows you to feel positive about yourself and your caregiving abilities. Group members often provide each other with a strong sense of togetherness and ongoing support. Participants are often amazed to find out that their problems or feelings are not unique.

Reading literature on aspects of Alzheimer's Disease allows caregivers to familiarize themselves with possible changes which may occur in the individual's behavior. Through education about the disease, caregivers can more fully understand and perceive some of the special needs of their loved ones. This is especially important as the disease progresses and individuals are unable to communicate their needs or desires. For information on the closest chapter support group, contact your local Alzheimer's Association Chapter.

Devotional

The Lord commanded Moses to go to Pharaoh and demand the release of the Hebrew slaves. What a difficult assignment! Moses was just a shepherd who had fled his country. Pharaoh was the ruthless leader of the world's most powerful nation, and the slaves were a vital part of the Egyptian economy.

You can understand why Moses experienced self-doubt. He protested to God: "I can't do that! Pharaoh won't pay any attention to me . . . I'm not a good speaker . . . Please send someone else."

Moses had one objection after another, but God continued to reassure Moses: "I'll be with you . . . I'll provide miracles to persuade Pharaoh . . . I'll tell you what to say . . . Now go!"

When Moses trusted God and obeyed, he was able to accomplish the tasks. In fact, Moses became even more powerful and famous than Pharaoh.

You have a difficult assignment. Caring for an Alzheimer's patient can be tedious, thankless, exasperating, demanding and unrelenting. But with God's help you can do much more than you ever imagined.

God's resources are unlimited. He will reinforce you and give you the daily manna you need to be sustained. "God is able to do immeasurably more than all we ask or imagine according to His power that is at work in us" (Ephesians 3:20).

LONELINESS

S ince my wife was first diagnosed with Alzheimer's Disease my whole life has seemed so empty. I miss the conversations that we used to have about our children, our shared interests. She can no longer remember conversations that we've had just moments earlier. I know there may come a day when she won't even remember me.

Practical Suggestions

Loneliness may occur as a feeling of being without companionship or as being cut off from others. When unresolved, loneliness can decrease one's ability to function and may increase social isolation.

There are many variables that can enhance the feeling of loneliness. The most common is the gradual decline of personal contact with family and friends. Predisposing factors, including loss of companionship, increased caregiver responsibilities, role reversal, and the increased emotional toll of caregiving, put the caregiver at greater risk for experiencing a sense of isolation. In some support groups that I have facilitated, many caregivers have expressed a sense of fear of the unknown, as well as a sense of doom about the future. Caregivers need to be encouraged to take time out to relieve themselves of the constant demands placed upon them. Make an attempt to have at least two activities outside your home each week.

Involvement in activities and social networking allow you to meet other people who share similar interests. Social support opportunities can allow the caregiver to perceive and believe that he or she can obtain support or a listening ear whenever they truly need one.

Community services including in-home respite and adult day care are available as alternative resources. Caregivers should be aware that they are at a much greater risk of burn-out if they isolate themselves from others. Respite care can be an invaluable resource in sharing the care needs of the memory-impaired person.

Devotional

A good marriage is the deepest relationship known to man. In the beginning God said, "It is not good that Man is alone." He caused a deep sleep to come upon Adam, took a rib from his side and created a woman to be his companion. God could have created Woman from the dust of the ground, but instead He created Eve from Adam's rib to demonstrate the closeness of the marital relationship.

A respected minister said, "God took a bone from Adam's side to create Eve. He did not take a bone from his head so that she would rule over him, or a bone from his foot that she would be under him. God took a bone from his side that she would be next to him, from next to his heart that he might love her and from under his arm that he might protect her."

Much of the loneliness you now feel is caused by the erosion of an intimate relationship. It is similar to the loneliness one feels when a mate dies. In fact, until a cure is found, there is a sense in which Alzheimer's Disease takes a person's life by degrees. You are beginning to experience the loss of a loved one, but without the support and sympathy most people receive when a loved one dies.

Those who have not experienced what you are enduring can't possibly understand how devastating it is to come to the realization that you are living with a person who is different than the one who was your daily companion.

That is why it is imperative that you deepen your spiritual life during this trial, that you develop meaningful relationships and enjoyable activities outside the home, and that you inter-act with others who have had similar experiences. No one understands like those who have been there. The Bible says, "Though one may be overpowered, two can defend themselves. A cord of three strands is not quickly broken (Ecclesiastes 4:12).

WANDERING

Most of my time is spent making sure that my wife doesn't wander out of our house. Her ability to retrace her way and find rooms in our home is becoming more and more of a challenge. I fear for the worst and worry about what might happen to her if she gets out. She can no longer say who she is, let alone where she lives.

Practical Suggestions

As Alzheimer's Disease progresses, the individual loses the ability to retrace a directional way back home. There are many reasons why an Alzheimer's patient wanders or walks away from home.

It is important to assess and determine the possible reasons for this behavior. Is there something that has happened that may have triggered the wandering episode? Explore possible causes such as medications; external stimuli such as noise; fear or restlessness; and the need to meet basic requirements including hunger and toiletry.

Be aware that wandering behavior may follow a specific pattern or trend. Is there a particular time of day or night that the individual has a tendency to wander? Has there been any previous history or episodes of wandering that may give you a clue as to whether there is an intended destination?

Household areas that appear safe to you as a caregiver may not be for the individual with Alzheimer's Disease. Safety precautions such as door locks or curtains covering the handle need to be established as individuals become at risk for wandering out of their homes. Consider hedges or a fence with a locked gate as an additional security measure. When used properly, household safety devices can deter wandering and alert the caregiver to this potential risk.

As a preventive measure, keep a recent portrait photo of the affected individual on file. This could assist law enforcement officers and the media in locating your loved one should he or she wander away from home.

Devotional

Sometimes the Lord uses our difficult personal experiences to teach us valuable spiritual lessons. When someone you love wanders away and endangers himself or herself, it illustrates how frustrating it must be for God when we wander from Him.

The Bible says, "We all, like sheep, have gone astray, each of us has turned to his own way" (Isaiah 53:6). Sheep are not very smart animals. They cannot protect themselves and they cannot find their way home, yet they insist on wandering away from their shepherd. But the good shepherd will seek after a lost, confused sheep and lovingly carry it back to the fold.

Just as you make every effort to protect your loved one from harming himself, so God endeavors to protect us from the consequences of our own sin. Just as you lovingly pursue the one who wanders off, so the Lord pursues those who stray from Him. And just as you tenderly, kindly bring the wanderer home, so God seeks to bring us back to Himself.

Jesus said, "Suppose one of you has a hundred sheep and loses one of them. Does he not leave the ninety-nine in the open country and go after the lost sheep until he finds it? And when he finds it, he joyfully puts it on his shoulders and goes home. Then he calls his friends and neighbors together and says, 'Rejoice with me; I have found my lost sheep.' I tell you that in the same way there will be more rejoicing in heaven over one sinner who repents than over ninety-nine righteous persons who do not need to repent" (Luke 15:4-7).

GUILT

*L*ately *when I've gone out to take care of some personal business, I've felt guilty for having left my husband alone. It seems that when he's with me, it takes me an awfully long time to get the things done that I need to do. I just don't know what to do! I really miss his not being able to go with me. We used to take short rides around town just to enjoy being together. Now, he can't even sit still for a short ride.*

Practical Suggestions

Guilt is often associated with the feeling that you have done something wrong. Usually, guilt is indicative of feeling inadequate or having not done enough.

One of the most difficult dilemmas facing caregivers is the need to protect the individual from personal injury or making decisions based upon his or her poor judgment. This often entails reducing the freedom of the person to actively participate in making decisions, and may cause an uneasiness on the part of the caregiver.

The transition of responsibilities from one marriage partner to the other can be complicated. This is especially true in the early stages of the disease when the impaired individual is still able to project feelings of guilt on the caregiver. Role reversal often requires that you reassure yourself that you are doing all that you can under the present circumstances.

Many caregivers I've spoken to have expressed an initial feeling of anxiety but were comfortable with their decisions once they acted upon them. It may be helpful to seek out family and friends for their personal support and continued friendship. Remember, as a caregiver, you also must take care of your spiritual, physical and emotional needs.

13

Devotional

Jiminy Cricket used to sing, "Always let your conscience be your guide." But the conscience is not always a reliable guide. The conscience is often like a computer, giving out what it has been programmed to compute. There was an old computer slogan — GIGO — which stands for "Garbage in, garbage out." You can program your conscience to guide you in the wrong direction if you are not careful. The Bible speaks of several different kinds of consciences. Hebrews 10:22 speaks of a **guilty conscience** — one that has violated God's commands and appropriately feels guilty because it **is** guilty. Then there is a **seared conscience** (I Timothy 4:2), which has been violated so often that it no longer feels guilty even when it should feel guilty. The I.R.S. has a conscience fund to which violators can send in cash anonymously to relieve their guilt. One man sent in $150 with a note that read, "I failed to pay what I should have; if my conscience still hurts me, I'll send in the rest."

The Bible also mentions a **weak conscience** (I Corinthians 8:10), which has been programmed to believe that certain activities are sinful when they are not. An anorexic may feel guilty when eating, but the guilt is from a weak, falsely programmed conscience.

Then there is a **good conscience** (I Peter 3:21), which has been cleansed through obedience to Christ and which lives a righteous life without guilt.

In a good marriage the conscience has been programmed to share nearly everything with the marriage partner. When Alzheimer's Disease strikes and necessity dictates that the sharing be reduced, it is natural to experience some guilt feelings. But the guilt comes from a weak conscience that must now be reprogrammed to understand that the circumstances have changed. What once would have been considered selfish behavior is now in the best interest of the marriage. The relationship is entering a new phase which will require less intimacy and more independence.

"Let us draw near to God with a sincere heart in full assurance of faith, having our hearts sprinkled to cleanse us from a guilty conscience and having our bodies washed with pure water" (Hebrews 10:22).

EMBARRASSMENT
(UNDRESSING)

M*ary and I used to visit our friends quite a lot. Lately though, she has been disrobing in public places. Without warning, she'll begin taking off her clothing. It really has been quite embarrassing — especially the time we were at the shopping mall. I just don't know what to do. I've tried buying her clothing that snaps in the back, but somehow she figures out how to get that undone, too.*

Practical Suggestions

As Alzheimer's Disease progresses societal norms that have been learned are now forgotten. The individual's judgment may become impaired to the point that he or she forgets how to properly dress themselves. The person may take clothing that is uncomfortable off in public without even realizing what he or she has done.

The caregiver should attempt to use distraction or diversion when the individual undresses inappropriately. Undressing may be a sign or clue that the individual is uncomfortable or anxious. Be sure to assess whether there is a specific reason for the individual's behavior. The person may feel uncomfortable in their clothing or their behavior may be indicative of some other need such as toiletry or rest.

Caregivers can alter clothing garments using special zippers or buttons that make it difficult to undress Remember, the caregiver often becomes more upset and embarrassed regarding the incident than the individual. Attempt to keep your emotions in perspective.

Devotional

In Luke 8:35 we read that Jesus encountered an uncontrollable man whose behavior was barbarous. The man would run naked through the local cemetery, terrorizing the people. When Jesus healed the man of his demon possession, the people were amazed at the transformation that occured. "And the people went out to see what had happened. When they came to Jesus, they found the man from whom the demons had gone out, sitting at Jesus' feet, dressed and in his right mind" (Luke 8:35). Note that when the man was in his right mind he immediately clothed himself.

Even today when a person's mind begins to wane he will often lose concern about his clothing and appearance. It probably has nothing to do with demon possession, but everything to do with a loss of clear thinking. When you are embarrassed by a loved one attempting to disrobe at an inappropriate time, remember several things: Your loved one is not in his or her right mind; his indiscretion is not a reflection on you or the care you are giving; what others think is not all that important (compassionate people understand and the rest don't matter); God sees His people completely clothed in His righteousness and the embarrassment of our sin is completely covered at all times.

"I delight greatly in the Lord; my soul rejoices in my God. For he has clothed me with garments of salvation and arrayed me in a robe of righteousness" (Isaiah 61:10).

INCONTINENCE

T his disease is really beginning to take its toll on my husband. He can no longer take care of his personal needs and he has become so much like a child. He relieves himself wherever the urge leads him. Of all the aspects of this disease, his inability to take care of his personal needs seems to upset me the most. He was always so particular about the way he looked and dressed, always wanting to be so perfect.

Practical Suggestions

Urinary incontinence is one of the major reasons Alzheimer's patients are placed in nursing homes. Some studies have indicated that incontinence may even affect one's functional independence.

Incontinence may occur due to forgetfulness rather than the individual's ability to control his or her bodily discharges. The problem occurs because the brain can't tell the individual fast enough that he or she needs to urinate.

Record keeping can assist the caregiver with identifying specific toiletry patterns or trends. Keep a notebook available and log the time of day, where, and the approximate amount the patient urinates. This tracking activity may identify appropriate time periods in which you may want to remind the individual to use the bathroom. Taking the individual to the bathroom on a regular basis may have some positive outcome on reducing incontinence.

The inability to locate the bathroom due to one's confusion also could be the source of concern. Illustrations placed on the bathroom door can assist the individual in finding the bathroom.

Caregivers should be sensitive not to punish failure or inappropriate urination. Instead, praise the individual when there is successful performance and be sure to dress the person in clothing that he or she easily can undo when necessary. Caregivers are especially challenged when attempting to balance the best approach to a person who is incontinent and also undresses in public.

Bathroom safety should also be a strong consideration. Install various safety features such as grab bars and non-skid rugs. The bathroom is one of the most dangerous areas for patient falls.

Devotional

An oil investor visited a leper colony while on a business trip in the Mideast. There he witnessed a dedicated missionary on her knees binding up the open, ulcerating wounds of a leper. The sight was so repulsive that the businessman turned away and said in disgust, "I would not do that for a million dollars."

The missionary overheard him. Compassionately but frankly, she replied, "Sir, neither would I."

People do things out of love that they would never do for money. Taking care of an Alzheimer's patient sometimes requires the performance of loathsome and abhorrent tasks. You could not be paid enough money to do what you are called upon to do. But you do it for love; you do it for your mate; you do it for Jesus Christ.

"Dear friends, do not be surprised at the painful trial you are suffering, as though something strange were happening to you. But rejoice that you participate in the suffering of Christ" (I Peter 4:12-13).

ABANDONMENT
(FAMILY)

After years of taking care of our children I feel
so abandoned. They no longer come around
as they used to now that their mother is in
the condition that she's in. When they do, their
visits are so short I feel as though they've visited
just long enough to say they were here. Why can't
they realize that I need them now more than ever?
I really miss their support and encouragement.

Practical Suggestions

Have you ever noticed how people handle emergency situations? There always seem to be those that remain calm and collected and those that lose control. Witnessing a loved one go through behavioral changes such as those exhibited by Alzheimer's patients reminds me of how people deal with emergencies.

Some people are able to deal openly with the illness while others feel uncomfortable. How we handle these delicate situations often depends on the types of defense mechanisms to which we've grown accustomed. Sometimes people act in a way that hurts you. This behavior isn't always because they don't care or love you; rather, it's their way of dealing with a sensitive issue.

Caregivers should openly discuss personal concerns and sensitive issues with family members. They may not fully understand the level of added responsibilities and personal needs that you are facing.

It is important that family members be supportive of each other during these difficult times. Attempting to force visitation and contact with the affected individual may only lead to further distancing. If appropriate, identify activities with which your family can assist you, but which don't require custodial care or a lot of "hands on" responsibilities.

Devotional

In a recent movie, the main character Forrest Gump is told repeatedly, "Run, Forrest, run!" Whenever Forrest faces a difficult challenge, he escapes by running away.

Most people tend to run away when they are frightened. They don't know how to respond, or they feel helpless in facing difficult circumstances, so they avoid them altogether. But sometimes running away leaves the courageous, responsible people behind to meet the challenges alone.

When Jesus was arrested and sent to trial, He certainly needed His disciples — His friends — with Him. But in His hour of greatest need, "Everyone deserted Him and fled" (Mark 14:50). Jesus faced His toughest battle alone. With His friends nowhere to be found, He endured a phony trial, false accusations, brutal beatings and a painful crucifixion.

But when Jesus rose from the grave, instead of condemning His disciples as cowards and alienating them even further, He patiently sought redemption. He did not demand an apology from His disciples. He welcomed their companionship and the relationships were immediately restored.

If family members let you down when you need them, you may want to tactfully communicate your concern. But then don't criticize them any further. Don't manipulate or threaten them. Don't alienate them. Be as understanding as possible. They will admire your patience and in the end they will be much more likely to return and assist you.

"To this you were called, because Christ suffered for you, leaving you an example, that you should follow in His steps" (I Peter 2:21).

DISTRESS
(NEW RESPONSIBILITIES)

O n the outside, I appear to be handling Bill's illness very well. On the inside, however, I'm emotionally stressed out. I feel the weight of the world coming down on me. There are so many things that I need to take over now. What do I know about finances, home repairs, and all the other things that I took for granted? Each day becomes a new challenge for me to keep things running smoothly.

Practical Suggestions

Most of the four million Americans diagnosed with Alzheimer's Disease are cared for in their homes and not in long term care facilities. If the ultimate goal is to maintain the individual in his or her home setting for as long as possible, it is essential that the caregiver take care of his or her own physical and emotional well-being.

Emotional and mental distress associated with caregiving is quite common. Recognize these feelings and set priorities for those activities or areas with which you feel uncomfortable. Caregivers almost invariably turn to their families for support and respite. Sometimes, however, these support systems are not adequate or available, so the need for outside resources becomes essential. Explore the available resources and services in your area that can assist you with unfamiliar activities. Seek guidance from family or friends about the steps necessary to overcome and resolve problem areas. Usually a referral about a reputable repair person or an accountant can be an enormous help.

Often, it is not a financial barrier preventing caregivers from obtaining services, but rather a distrust of strangers providing care, as well as concerns about quality and providers' experience.

If you are considering the use of outside agencies, there are a few steps to consider. Begin by identifying the services you need and when these services would be of the most help to you. Evaluate local service providers through your own Alzheimer's network. The local chapter is an excellent resource to provide you with names and references of families who have already used agency services.

Once you engage in using outside help, be sure to provide clear instructions regarding caregiving approaches. Caregivers are often more knowledgeable about specific interventions that work in delicate situations. Adjustments to the presence of a new caregiver often will take some time for your loved one.

Lastly, develop an ongoing process of evaluation. With time, a good service provider should be able to adjust to the specific needs of the Alzheimer's patient, realizing that no single provider can meet all of their personal needs.

Devotional

A wise country philosopher once said, "If you have a frog to swallow, don't look at it very long. And if you have more than one frog to swallow, swallow the big one first!"

A lot of wisdom is contained in that homespun counsel. When you face an unpleasant challenge, don't spend a lot of time fretting over it. Once you realize what needs to be done, go to work. Worrying only makes your challenge appear even more difficult than it really is. When you begin working, you will gain the confidence needed to complete your assignment.

If you have several large tasks to perform, tackle the largest one first to get it out of the way. Don't be too proud to ask a competent person to help you. Once you have conquered the biggest challenge, you will know that, with the Lord's help, you can do the rest.

Jesus said, "But seek first His kingdom and His righteousness, and all these things will be given to you as well" (Matthew 6:33).

SUFFERING
(INJURIES)

M ary can no longer tell me what hurts or bothers her. Today, she tripped over a stool that's been in the same place for years. Her arms and legs are pretty bruised up, yet she doesn't say a word. I feel helpless that she's in so much pain and I can't do anything.

Practical Suggestions

The home environment is filled with potentially harmful areas and hazards which can pose significant risks of injury to a person with Alzheimer's Disease. Altered vision, hearing, touch and the ability to recognize temperature sensitivity are all factors that increase the possibility of an accident.

Through the use of an organized home safety assessment tool, caregivers can identify and correct personal and environmental risk factors associated with injuries. As Alzheimer's Disease progresses, the caregiver's ability to anticipate and perceive safety needs becomes a crucial role. When considering safety assessments, the caregiver should attempt to recognize problems while they are still just potential problems.

Prevention is essential to reducing or eliminating personal injuries. Assess each room of your household for potential dangers. Remember, what might be safe for you may not be for someone with a cognitive impairment such as Alzheimer's Disease.

Special consideration should be given to the bathroom, bedroom and kitchen. These rooms can have multiple hazards present, which can lead to fires, falls, scaldings, poisonings, electric shocks and drownings. Passageways need to be free from electrical cords, telephone extension cords or other potential hazards to prevent falls. Throw rugs should be eliminated wherever possible.

Devotional

It is painful to see someone you love hurting. The Bible says that the family of God is like a body — when one part suffers we all suffer with it. It is natural for you to want to do everything you can to prevent your loved one from experiencing pain.

If God really loves us, why does He allow us to suffer at all? If He is all-powerful, why doesn't He just eliminate the pain? The question of human suffering has plagued theologians since the time of Job.

The first chapter of II Corinthians suggests several reasons why God permits suffering. According to this passage, we experience pain for the following reasons: to identify with Christ's sufferings (verse 5); to develop patience (verse 6); to receive God's comfort (verse 9); and to witness to others about our faith (verse 11).

While the problem of suffering is perplexing, one thing is clear: when we endure pain ourselves, we are better equipped to minister to others who hurt. God "comforts us in all our troubles, so that we can comfort those in any trouble with the comfort we ourselves have received" (II Corinthians 1:4).

I once giggled at a friend of mine who was writhing in pain from a kidney stone. "It's not as serious as it appears," I flippantly assured him. "It's just a kidney stone. You'll pass it and be perfectly healthy in a few days." I was right.

But then one night I awakened with an excruciating pain in my back. I felt as if someone had stabbed me with a knife! I was diagnosed as having a kidney stone. I passed it the next day and have been healthy ever since. But now I don't smile when I hear someone has a kidney stone. I am **very** sympathetic! Because I empathize, instead of laughing I try to comfort the one who is suffering.

In the midst of your painful experience remember that even Jesus suffered, and he was a perfect man. But if you will hold on to your faith there will come a day when God will use your hurt to comfort someone else. No one understands like someone who has been there.

LETTING GO

> **M**y husband is no longer the person I married. This disease has robbed him of his personality many years ago. I see in him a skeletal reminder of a person who once was. It's so difficult for me to see him deteriorate like this. His life was so full of vigor and energy.

Practical Suggestions

Caregivers may go through a sense of mourning and loss even though their loved one is still physically alive. The progressive nature of this disease may often put the caregiver on an emotional roller coaster: one moment hope, the next despair.

How discouraging it is to observe families who are given a false sense of hope when they temporarily witness a positive change in their loved one's behavior. This ongoing battle of not knowing when the individual will take a step for the worse is agonizing for the caregiver and his or her family.

Compounding the problem is the fact that no two people exhibit the same behaviors in the exact time frame. Attempts by caregivers to compare notes with other providers often result in disappointment.

It is important to know that caregivers experience a grief process during their caregiving roles. Adjustments to role reversals, as well as the loss of companionship with their partners, place additional stress and anxiety on caregivers.

A variety of strategies can help you cope with this loss. Attempt to keep busy and participate in social groups. Seeking professional help and guidance through support groups or other networks, such as your church or your local chapter of the Alzheimer's Association, can also provide you with the strength to move forward.

Devotional

A friend of mine looks at his life in terms of chapters. Chapter one was "preparation" when he received his education. Chapter two, "ministry," was when he served as a pastor of a local church. Chapter three was "teaching" — he was a professor in a seminary for several years. Now instead of retiring, he says he is moving into another chapter: "writing and lecturing."

What a great way to view life! Each chapter is different. Each has distinct challenges and opportunities. When one chapter ends, another begins.

Some people miss out on the privileges and excitement of today because they are still living in yesterday's chapter, pining for the past. Most likely they are exaggerating how good that chapter really was. Someone said, "Nostalgia isn't what it used to be!" But no one's life remains the same, so it is imperative that we learn to make every day count.

You are coming to the close of a very important chapter of your life. Many good things have happened and you will often review this chapter with fond memories. But it is time to bring this chapter of your life to a close and begin a new chapter. It will not be easy or without tears and grief, but it is possible.

Joining a support group could help make the transition easier. It is encouraging to share with others who have had similar experiences and have found joy in the next chapter of life.

"There is a time for everything, and a season for every activity under heaven: a time to be born and a time to die, a time to plant and a time to uproot, a time to kill and a time to heal, a time to tear down and a time to build, a time to weep and a time to laugh, a time to mourn and a time to dance" (Ecclesiastes 3:1-4).

FIDGETING

Mary has become more preoccupied with buttoning and unbuttoning her clothes. The other day I watched her zip and unzip her sweater no telling how many times. It's as though she has this wound up energy and she has no knowledge as to how to best use it. I'm a little concerned about this behavior being misinterpreted as craziness or some other weird thing.

Practical Suggestions

As Alzheimer's Disease progresses, you may begin to observe an individual's restless movements such as tying and untying knots, fidgeting with buttons on his or her clothing and playing with zippers. This behavior is often characterized by increased motor activity and restless movements. Fidgeting may indicate that the person has some degree of discomfort and may warrant assessment on the part of the caregiver.

Common reasons for this behavior are that clothing may be too tight or too warm for the individual. Thoroughly assess the possible causes for this behavior and be sensitive to increased external stimulation. I normally suggest that the caregiver evaluate events that may have recently changed in the person's environment, as these might be causing this behavior.

Often, increased noise or traffic during visitation has a tendency to overload the person and results in this restless activity. If necessary, move the individual away from these activities or limit the amount of contact he or she has with visitors.

Sometimes this behavior occurs due to the disease process and not something that is taking place in the environment. When necessary, the caregiver should attempt to use diversion or distraction as a means to eliminate this behavior.

Devotional

The Bible says that God leads His people like an eagle teaches her young to fly: ". . . like an eagle that stirs up its nest and hovers over its young, that spreads its wing to catch them and carries them on it pinions" (Deuteronomy 32:11).

It must be frightening to learn how to fly. Even a baby eagle must want to stay in the nest where it is safe and secure. In Biblical times there was a type of eagle that had a strange custom for teaching its young to fly. The mother eagle would first stir up the nest, taking out the things that made the nest soft and cozy. Suddenly the baby eagles would be pricked with sticks and briars and, unable to get comfortable, would want out of the nest.

Next the mother eagle would "hover over its young," demonstrating how to fly. Then she would place a baby eagle on her wings, carry it hundreds of feet into the air, then turn over, forcing the eaglet to learn to fly as he falls. If the baby eagle didn't learn on the first trip, she would swoop down to catch him. What a trip! Can't you just picture the terrified, bug-eyed baby eagle, clutching onto its mother's back, pleading, "Is this trip really necessary?" But through that trauma the eagle quickly learned how to fly and was never again satisfied with just staying in the nest.

God leads us like that. Sometimes when we get too comfortable with our situation, He stirs up our nest and we get restless. Most of us tend to get too comfortable with this world. We settle down and feel cozy here. We forget that God has a higher calling for us in heaven. God sometimes stirs up our nest to remind us that "This world is not my home, I'm just passin' through."

When you witness your loved one fidgeting or restless, consider it a positive sign — spiritually. God is stirring up his nest. Your loved one is getting ready to move on to a higher existence, to get out of this nest and fly!

FAITH
(TRUST)

W ho would have ever thought that I'd be placed in this position called caregiver? This disease is so unforgiving, so devastating. I always felt so secure knowing that my wife could give me the kind of advice I needed in a pinch. My prayers are now focused on making it through this ordeal. I've asked myself a thousand times, Why me, Lord? Why us? I must keep faith that somehow I will grow stronger through this ordeal and through the challenges ahead.

Practical Suggestions

Caregiving tests one's faith. Initially upon diagnosis, many caregivers express a strong sense of "Why me, Lord?" There is an attempt to fully understand how and why their loved one has been dealt such a devastating future. After weeks and months of soul searching, the answer becomes clear. There is a realization that you didn't do anything that could have changed the circumstances. How you respond to being a caregiver, however, can mean the difference in the individual's ability to deal and cope with this disease. Continued loyalty and faithfulness to your loved one will be challenged daily. The days ahead will sometimes be difficult and hard to understand.

Many caregivers have expressed the meaningfulness of prayer during the difficult times of providing for the needs of their loved ones. Visitation from your clergy member may provide you with support and an outlet for spiritual expression and growth.

Devotional

Billy Graham once told about a circus entertainer who dazzled a huge crowd by walking across a tightrope above Niagara Falls. When he was finished, the crowd burst into applause. He then walked back across the wire, pushing an empty wheelbarrow. Again the audience cheered in approval.

"How many of you believe I could push a person in the wheelbarrow across the falls?" the entertainer asked. Several hands went up. Pointing to a young man in the front row, the tightrope walker asked, "Do you really believe I could put a man in this wheelbarrow and push him across?"

"Yes, sir!" the boy exclaimed.

"OK," said the entertainer, "Get in. You're first."

The boy couldn't be seen for the dust he left as he ran away!

It is one thing to say we believe in God; it's another to put our trust in Him when our security is at stake. But genuine faith still believes even when life is insecure and illogical.

Job said, "Though he slay me, yet will I hope in him" (Job 13:15). J. Oswald Sanders said that faith is willing to travel under sealed orders. Faith continues to trust God even though the future is uncertain.

Someone wrote, "Have faith in yourself and you are doomed to disappointment. Have faith in your friends and they will die and leave you. Have faith in money and you may have it taken from you. Have faith in reputation and some slanderous tongue may blast it. But have faith in God and you will never be disappointed in time or eternity, for Jesus never fails."

"And without faith it is impossible to please God, because anyone who comes to Him must believe that He exists and that He rewards those who earnestly seek Him" (Hebrews 11:6).

FEAR
(HEREDITARY)

The doctors say that there is a possibility of this disease being passed on to one of our children. I've thought about this issue a lot. Which one of the two? They both have so much to live for; how could this disease strike twice? I could see the fear in their eyes when they heard this from the doctor. Even if we knew, what could we do?

Practical Suggestions

Sometimes we are so overcome with fear that it begins to affect our daily lives and the way we function. We can become so preoccupied with the unknown that we begin to self destruct.

The diagnosis of any major illness can have a numbing effect on the individual and his or her family. When the disease, such as Alzheimer's, has no known cause or cure, the concern regarding heredity can become overwhelming for other family members.

Researchers are extensively investigating the possible causes of Alzheimer's Disease and are beginning to discover some common factors or traits. Unfortunately, these efforts have not yet singled out a cause or led to a cure.

Family members are encouraged to thoroughly discuss their concerns about hereditary factors with their family physicians. Have you ever felt bad and were hesitant to have a medical evaluation? Remember the level of anxiety and fear that you went through? If your family has concerns about this issue, don't delay.

Help is available through the Alzheimer's Association and other fine health service providers. They are excellent resources for current research information.

Devotional

It has been said that worry is the act of enjoying a crisis before it occurs. Three times in the Sermon on the Mount Jesus commanded, "Do not worry" (Matthew 6:24-34). He said that if God provides food for the birds of the air and clothing for the lilies of the field, then He will provide for the needs of His people.

There is a significant difference between being concerned and being worried. Concern focuses on probable difficulties and results in action. We ought to be concerned about the future enough to prepare for it. Jesus said, "No man builds a tower without first sitting down and calculating the cost." Concern motivates us to buy life insurance, install smoke detectors, save for college tuition and get annual physicals.

But anxiety focuses on uncontrollable circumstances and produces inaction. Worry always asks, "What if"? What if there is an earthquake? What if the economy collapses? What if the plane crashes? What if my child suffers from Alzheimer's Disease also?

Worry is a waste of time. "Who of you by worrying can add a single hour to his life?" (Matthew 6:27). Worry doesn't extend your life — it actually reduces life expectancy. It's counterproductive.

Worry is also a sin. Worry calls God a liar. God's Word says, "in all things God works for the good of those who love Him . . ." (Romans 8:28). The person who worries is communicating that he doesn't think God will keep that promise.

Worry is also a thief. It robs us of the joy of today by forcing us to focus on the fears of tomorrow. Jesus encouraged us to learn the art of living one day at a time. "Therefore do not worry about tomorrow, for tomorrow will worry about itself. Each day has enough trouble of its own" (Matthew 6:34).

Tomorrow will have problems, but God will give you the resources to meet them. Focus on the blessings of today. Say with the Psalmist, "This is the day that the Lord has made, let us rejoice and be glad in it!" (Psalm 118:24).
Said the robin to the sparrow,

"I would really like to know
Why those anxious human beings
Rush about and worry so."
Said the sparrow to the robin,
"I think that it must be
That they have no heavenly Father
Such as cares for you and me."

COMPANIONSHIP

I miss the personal companionship that I had with my wife. I know deep down inside that she's there somewhere. If I could only find a way to connect with her to tell her how much I still love her, to let her know I'll be there until the end. Somehow when I look into her eyes, I think she knows.

Practical Suggestions

Of all of the issues expressed to me by caregivers in support groups, the loss of spousal companionship is by far the most difficult for them to discuss. Somehow, society has stereotyped the elderly into hiding their affection and sexual feeling for each other.

I recall the time one woman discussed her need to be affectionately touched by her husband and questioned whether this was right or appropriate. There was a strong sense of guilt and shame on her part for still loving her husband and wanting to be intimately involved with him after twenty-seven years of marriage. We discussed alternative options to meet her emotional needs.

Expressing one's love through closeness and touch is often a good means of communicating to the individual suffering from Alzheimer's Disease. Non-verbal communication is an essential means of getting your message across.

The expression of love through touch can have a therapeutic effect with no further desire than the enjoyment of the physical presence of your mate. Evaluate the individual's comfort level and be cautious not to frighten them.

Devotional

On August 4, 1993, our local newspaper carried the touching story about Matt Ross, an elementary student in Owensboro,

Kentucky, who was returning to school after receiving six weeks of treatments in his battle against leukemia. He had lost all his hair, so he donned his favorite baseball cap and headed for school, very concerned about the reaction of his classmates. Would they gawk and make fun of his bald head? Would he be isolated because he now looked so different?

When Matt arrived he found five of his friends wearing baseball caps, too. They removed their caps to show Matt that all five of them had shaved their heads. "We just wanted Matt to know he had friends," they said (*Courier-Journal*, August 4, 1993).

There are many non-verbal ways to express love: a smile, a thoughtful gift, a wink . . . even a shaved head! But one of the most effective ways to express love is through physical touch.

Jesus often communicated love through physical touch. People in Jesus's time were often repulsed by lepers because they were highly contagious and the disease made a person appear grotesque. (People today may shun AIDS patients or even those with noncontagious diseases like Alzheimer's). But Jesus "reached out and touched" a leper and said, "Be clean" (Matthew 8:3).

When the disciples were afraid, Jesus touched them to calm their fears (Matthew 17:7). His compassion for two blind men drove Him to touch their eyes and give them sight (Matthew 20:34).

Though your touch is not accompanied by miraculous healings, you have the power to communicate love through a compassionate arm about the shoulder, a gentle pat on the arm or a tender touch on the face. Often these expressions of love are accepted and understood when verbal expressions cannot be comprehended.

DISTANCE
(PERSONAL)

Isn't it ironic that I'm now having to take care of my mother? We were never really close; in fact, I resented her for spending more time with my brother. Now I must care for her every need. I pray that I'll be able to reconcile with my feelings toward her. One thing is for sure with this disease: it's been able to bring two people together after so many years of being apart.

Practical Suggestions

Adult children are providing more attention and care for their elderly parents than ever before. Role reversal is a difficult challenge at best. When it happens to be with a parent, it may bring a lifelong agenda of unresolved issues.

Financial strains, lifestyle changes and emotions of guilt can complicate an already poor relationship. Conflictual issues such as the loss of the parent's parenting role, the parent-child relationship and the parent's presence in the adult child's home can also strain this new responsibility.

If necessary, seek guidance and direction from someone close to you. Remember that, just as it takes time to build good relationships, it also takes time to mend and heal bad ones. Allow yourself time to adequately adjust to this new life experience. Through talking, you can move toward solving problems.

Devotional

The Western world has brainwashed us to believe that love is primarily an emotion. Think of the popular songs in recent years that have communicated that idea. A few decades ago we heard, "Some enchanted evening, you will meet a stranger

. . . across a crowded room . . ." According to the song, some-how, someday your knees will wobble and your heart will pound and you will have fallen in love!

Then Elvis sang, "I can't help falling in love with you." That was followed by the Righteous Brothers, who whined, "You've lost that lovin' feelin!" The worst example came from the rock group The Doors when they sang "Hello, I love you, won't you tell me your name?"

But real love is not just a romantic feeling. Love means doing the right thing regardless of emotion. It is wonderful when love is accompanied by positive feelings, but emotions fluctuate. Sometimes loving feelings aren't there. Unconditional love (the Bible calls it "agape") is a deliberate act of the will. The best synonym for this God-like love is unselfishness. Unconditional love means making a conscious decision, regardless of feelings, to sacrifice your own selfish interests for the good of the other.

Maybe you don't have positive feelings toward the one entrusted to your care. That might change in time, but in a way it is irrelevant. Jesus did not feel like going to the cross for us. He prayed, "Father, if it be possible, let this cup pass from me." But He chose to be unselfish. "Nevertheless," he prayed, "not my will but thine be done."

"Greater love has no one than this, that he lay down his life for his friends" (John 15:13). To completely give up self for the good of the other — regardless of your feelings — is to show true love.

CLINGING

*M*y husband likes to follow me around the house. He's like my shadow, always right beside me. Sometimes it's very annoying because I need my own personal space. I can't even use the bathroom without him wanting to follow.

Practical Suggestions

In the early stages of Alzheimer's Disease, the individual is keenly able to mask and hide his or her difficulties. Defense mechanisms that are intact allow the individual to cover up mistakes. It is only as the disease progresses that the individual is no longer able to cover up these problems, bringing attention to the family that something is seriously wrong.

As persons' judgments become impaired, they begin to lose their sense of security with their surroundings. They gradually become more dependent on their caregivers. This dependency is often exhibited through what we call clinging behavior or shadowing.

Clinging behavior may represent familiarity and security to the individual suffering from Alzheimer's Disease. Caregivers should maintain consistency in their home environment, as the individual is better able to handle structured routines.

Activities should be consistent from day to day. Deviation from the normal routines of household schedules may cause the individual to exhibit increased symptoms of clinging, restlessness and even agitation.

This behavior often occurs as a result of the person being unable to process all of the external stimuli. If this should happen, simply remove the person from the activity.

Devotional

Jesus occasionally had a difficult time getting away from people. When he learned that his cousin and friend John the

Baptist had been killed by King Herod, "Jesus, withdrew by boat privately to a solitary place" (Matthew 14:13). He wanted to be alone with His closest friends in a time of grief and anger.

But the Bible says that the crowds, when they heard where he had gone, ran around the lake to meet Him on the other side! Imagine traveling across a large lake, anticipating a time of privacy and rest, only to be greeted on the other side of the lake by a mob of demanding people waving and smiling at you from the shore! Jesus's disciples must have said, "No! Not more people! We have had it up to here with people!" But, when Jesus landed and saw a large crowd, he had compassion on them and healed their sick (Matthew 14:14).

All day long Jesus ministered to those people. "As evening approached, the disciples came to Him and said, 'This is a remote place, and it's already getting late. Send the crowds away, so they can go to the villages and buy themselves some food" (Matthew 14:15). Doesn't that sound like something we would say? "It's time to quit. These thoughtless people came all the way around the lake without bringing a lunch. They are leeches! Send them home!"

Jesus suggested that they feed the people themselves. He then took one boy's small lunch and multiplied the five biscuits and two fish into enough food to feed over five thousand people. Jesus was amazing. Not only could he perform miracles, but he had the energy and the compassion to minister to people no matter how demanding they might become.

It is emotionally draining to have someone constantly following you, making demands on your time. It is normal to get exasperated. Pray for the patience and energy that Jesus Christ exemplified. Ephesians 3:16 is a good prayer: "I pray that out of His glorious riches He may strengthen you with power through His Spirit in your inner being."

While you pray for patience and energy, also remember the importance of an occasional time away from people. "Jesus often withdrew to lonely places and prayed" (Luke 5:16).

HOARDING

Today my wife was stopped by the mall security guard and accused of shoplifting. She had no idea what all the fuss was about. Her pockets were filled with goods, items she had no use for or would ever need. I've noticed lately at home that she has begun saving everything: old tissues, newspaper scraps. Her drawers are filled with this stuff.

Practical Suggestions

As the person's memory becomes more impaired, the individual may forget proper protocol when it comes to purchasing items. Instead of appropriately going through the checkout line, the individual may walk out not even realizing the action to be illegal.

The practice of collecting any number of things is one of the behavioral manifestations of Alzheimer's Disease. Hoarding items such as toilet tissue, paper clips, clothing, newspapers, etc., is another behavior that may be exhibited.

Many researchers believe that the hoarding or storing of material goods is associated with the individual's innate feeling of identity. "We are what we collect" is a phrase that comes to mind when I think of the many different objects patients have collected.

I've often thought that this behavior of collecting and hiding everything represents a sense of security and ownership for persons who otherwise are having difficulty in making daily decisions for themselves.

Caregivers should reinforce a sense of security with individuals who misplace things by assisting them with a search for their lost item(s). Another good way to reduce the chances of misplacing items is to reduce the number of possible hiding places by locking drawers, closets, cabinets and storage rooms.

Be careful to check clothes baskets and trash cans before

emptying. Family members should secure personal belongings such as jewelry and other valuable possessions in a locked box.

Caregivers should be alerted to the fact that the individual who hoards personal belongings may very well forget where they were placed and may become paranoid, believing that they have been stolen. False accusations to the police may result if the person seriously believes that someone, even you, has stolen their personal possessions.

Devotional

It may seem silly to us when someone finds security in accumulating trinkets and scraps from this world, but there is a sense in which we all do the very same thing. We all hoard things that are of no eternal value.

One evening on our vacation my family decided to play a game of Monopoly. It proved to be one of those rare nights for me. I was on a roll: On my first trip around the board I bought Indiana Avenue and Park Place. The next time around I landed on Kentucky Avenue and later Illinois Avenue and Boardwalk. I somehow acquired all four utilities. I could tell there was no stopping me!

Soon I began erecting houses and then hotels. My two sons kept complaining. "Dad, you are so lucky!" they whined. "That will be $400!" I would reply, hardly able to hide my smirk.

"I've got a hotel there. That will cost you $1,100!" I would say to the next customer. I accumulated hotels, deeds, houses and money. I was rich!

At about 1:00 a.m. the last survivor finally went bankrupt. I won! Each member of the family dejectedly got up from the table and headed for bed. I said, "Wait a minute! Someone needs to put away the game."

They kept walking and called back, "That's your reward for winning, Dad. It's all yours."

There I sat with all my loot. There was nothing left to do except scrape off the hotels and houses and put them in the box, along with my money and deeds. I closed the lid and headed upstairs to a cold bed.

My wife didn't say "I'm so proud of you! You were great tonight! You are Mr. Monopoly!" Instead she mumbled goodnight, rolled over and went to sleep! As I lay there in the darkness, I remembered Dr. James Dobson relating a similar experience and then comparing Monopoly to life. We work so hard to accumulate things so we can impress people who probably resent us anyway. Then one day we leave it all behind and stand before our Creator empty handed. What will matter then will not be our houses, gold, or land, but our character, our relationships with others and our salvation in Christ.

Only those who are not in their right mind find security in hoarding up things of this earth. That is why Jesus said, "Do not store up for yourselves treasures on earth, where moth and rust destroy, and where thieves break in and steal. But store up for yourselves treasures in heaven, where moth and rust do not destroy and where thieves do not break in and steal. For where your treasure is, there your heart will be also" (Matthew 6: 19:21).

Martyred missionary Jim Elliot said, "He is no fool who exchanges that which he cannot keep for that which he can never lose."

COMMUNICATION

Over a period of time my husband has had more difficulty understanding what I am saying to him. It's as though he grasps small pieces of my conversation but can't put the whole thing together. He replies with a lot of off-the-wall comments. His words make no sense or have no real meaning. I find myself having to repeat my statement over and over again. The more I try to clarify my comments, the more he becomes confused.

Practical Suggestions

The ability to communicate, both sending and receiving messages, is impaired in individuals suffering from Alzheimer's Disease. The inability to communicate is called aphasia. Thoughts are right at the tip of their tongues; however, trying to express and articulate them is another story.

When attempting to communicate, the caregiver should be calm and supportive. Maintain good eye contact with the person and use nonverbal clues such as hand gestures to support your message.

Sentences should be brief, using as few words as possible. Repeat the same statement over without restructuring your sentences. Often, parts of messages are received and it is necessary to repeat the exact message. Speak slowly and look directly at the individual when communicating.

The person with Alzheimer's Disease may unwittingly substitute the meaning of one word for another. Caregivers may be able to decode or decipher these words, allowing them to interpret the message. When the person uses the wrong word and you have been able to understand their intended word, reinforce the correct word. If this seems to bother or upset them then simply back off in your approach. Sometimes individuals can communicate through written notes and not verbal expressions. Explore this as an option when attempting to communicate.

Devotional

Perhaps the most important virtue for a compassionate caregiver is patience. To hear the same questions, to give the same answers, to deal with the same problems and to live with the same expressions of insecurity day after day is draining on one's nerves and energy.

In I Corinthians 13:4 patience is mentioned as the first quality of unconditional love. Patience is mentioned in Galatians 5:22 as one of the fruits of the Spirit. Someone said, "Patience is the ability to count down before blasting off!" The most popular prayer of Americans has probably been identified: "Lord, grant me patience — right now!"

My wife used to ride to work with the most patient man I have ever known. Oland Engle moved and talked slowly. He rarely drove over 45 miles an hour. He usually left 30 minutes early so he would not have to hurry. He was a patient listener who weighed every word carefully.

One day in heavy traffic an impetuous driver behind him honked the horn as soon as the light turned green. Oland moved on, but at the next light the same driver laid on the horn again. This time Oland put his car in park, got out, removed his pipe, slowly walked back to the driver, stooped down and asked, "Did you want something?"

"Yes," the stunned motorist said, "I'd like for you to get going."

"Well," Oland drawled, "if you hadn't blown the horn, I would have been gone by now!"

Anyone can lose patience. If you are weary of trying to communicate over and over again, pray for patience and remember how patient God has been with you.

GORGING

My husband's appetite has increased dramatically the last few months. No matter what he eats, it never seems to fill him up. Just the other day, we had finished dinner and it wasn't fifteen minutes before he asked me, "What's for dinner?"

Practical Suggestions

The overall nutritional goals for caregivers are to deter-mine the acceptable food preferences of the patient, to meet their nutritional needs and to figure out what approach works best in obtaining these objectives.

Functional loss due to memory impairment may signifi-cantly affect the person's dietary needs. They may have diffi-culty making choices from their plate and may even forget that they have just eaten.

Physical limitations may also present challenges to the patient. Swallowing and chewing may be difficult and the caregiver should be alert to the possibility of choking.

Loss of motor coordination may reduce the person's abil-ity to use utensils. Large-handled utensils or specially designed cups may assist individuals with picking up their food or hold-ing onto their drinks. A shortened attention span may indicate the need for small, more frequent feedings.

Store snacks such as chips and other goodies out of sight. Safety considerations for persons with memory impairment include kitchen appliances. Stoves or burners may be left on, creating a dangerous situation. Care also must be taken to prevent a patient from eating inedible items such as crayons, poisons, household plants, home decorations, etc. Secure your garbage can, as he or she may rummage through your trash and place table scraps back into the refrigerator, or even eat them. The caregiver should monitor the patient's food intake for proper nutritional balance.

Devotional

An insatiable appetite is a sign of a diseased mind. It is not normal for a person to desire food fifteen minutes after a sufficient meal. It would not be loving for a caregiver to continue to provide food on demand for one in that state of mind.

There are other kinds of inordinate appetites that are also unhealthy: the cravings for alcohol, prescription drugs, pornography or gambling can create addictions that will destroy the minds and bodies of ourselves and those we love.

But caring people refuse to allow the individual to continue the process of self-destruction. Although we cannot dictate every move another makes, love refuses to sit idly by while a friend is destroying himself. To speak up or take measures to help may require confrontation, intervention and frank communication, but love, "always protects" (I Corinthians 13:7).

The Bible says that because God loves us, "He will take pity on the weak and the needy and save the needy from death" (Psalm 72:13).

To an outsider it may appear cruel for you to refuse to allow the Alzheimer's patient to eat. It may appear condescending to hide the snacks, but in reality you are taking pity on the weak and saving them from premature death.

RIGIDITY

T his afternoon while I was watching television, I realized how much Ed had become like one of the characters. His robotic-like walk is so rigid and so stiff, as if it were not a free-flowing movement. I've noticed that his eyes rarely look down anymore when he's walking. His ability to get around the house is often restricted by small pieces of furniture. If I didn't keep these passageways clear, he'd be falling over them, oblivious to their presence.

Practical Suggestions

Disorders of posture, stance and movement become prominent as Alzheimer's Disease advances. Primary prevention should be aimed at keeping the individual as active and physically healthy as possible. There is definitely truth to the old saying "use it or lose it." Caregivers are strongly encouraged to actively engage the person in physical exercise, such as walks or activities that utilize different muscle groups.

It is easy to associate memory impairment with the inability to perform and maintain physical exercise. Consult with your physician if you feel uncomfortable about what your loved one can do in the way of activities.

Over time, you will begin to observe that the person's movements have become more rigid and stiff. Vision is usually focused forward with little attention being paid to peripheral objects or low-lying items. When this happens, the individual may become at risk for accidental falls.

The caregiver should attempt to remove small objects which may impede movement through passageways. Special attention should be made to areas like stairways and landings that pose a potential danger for falls.

Devotional

It can be discouraging to see what Alzheimer's does to the body. In fact there are many other diseases — cancer, heart disease, multiple sclerosis — that can attack and destroy our bodies. With all of these diseases there is a gradual (or even sometimes rapid) erosion of physical capabilities. The one who was once strong becomes weak. The one who was once alert becomes confused. The one who once stood erect is now stooped. The one who was once agile is now awkward and rigid.

It can be discouraging, but it should not be devastating. The Bible teaches: "Therefore, do not lose heart. Though outwardly we are wasting away, yet inwardly we are being renewed day by day. For our light and momentary troubles are achieving for us an eternal glory that far outweighs them all. So we fix our eyes not on what is seen, but on what is unseen. For what is seen is temporary, but what is unseen is eternal."

The obvious decaying of the body should remind us that our ultimate hope is not in what is physical, but what is spiritual. God promises to renew us within. He has promised that in heaven we will have new, eternal bodies that will never grow old. Though these diseases discourage us, they should not defeat us, because we focus "not on what is seen but what is unseen."

We've often sung, "When we've been there ten thousand years, bright shining as the sun, we've no less days to sing God's praise than when we first begun." Are those just words in a song that we have sung, or is it a truth we embrace? If eternity is true then we should not lose heart, even though outwardly we are wasting away. We believe that one day these troubles will seem to have lasted only a moment compared to an eternity of joy in heaven.

INFANTILIZATION

I must remember to allow my husband to do what he is capable of doing. I want so very much to help him that I often find myself doing everything for him. He's so capable of doing a lot of things for himself. This illness has robbed him of his mind, not his physical stamina or determination. At least not yet.

Practical Suggestions

When individuals are convinced that there is no use in responding to daily activities, they begin to experience feelings of apathy, hopelessness and a strong sense of dependency on others. Caregivers should encourage independence as long as possible.

It is often easier to do everything for the patient rather than allow them to do for themselves. Overprotective behavior is quite common among caregivers. Allow individuals to participate in activities of daily living and to do for themselves as much as possible without assistance.

Regular review and evaluation of specific activities should be done to ensure the ongoing safety of the individual. These areas may include using electrical appliances, mowing and other work-related activities.

If your loved one has problems staying on task, try different techniques that help get him or her refocused. Visually reinforce the task by demonstrating the activity. Sometimes, a simple start of the activity is all that is necessary for the individual to accomplish it. This is especially true with activities of daily living such as dressing or eating.

Also, remember to make decisions as easy as possible for the person. For example, laying the person's clothes out in sequential order may reduce the anxiety of trying to figure out which item goes on first.

Sensory overload and the need to make complicated decisions can cause extreme confusion, restlessness and agitation. Maintain independence as long as possible but limit activities that put unnecessary stress on the person.

Devotional

Have you ever watched a tiny baby chick peck its way out of a shell? It's a slow, exhausting process. You are tempted to break open the shell and let the pitiful, struggling creature go free. But you would not be helping the bird at all. The struggle to peck its way out of the shell stimulates the blood of the little creature, which is essential for the beginning of life. Without that struggle the baby chick would not live.

If you do for others what they can and should do for themselves, you will impede their growth and rob them of the challenges that are necessary for life. Overprotecting another is not an expression of love. It is usually an indication of our own desire to be needed or a sign of our impatience.

God loves us so much that He allows us (sometimes forces us) to struggle. He does not do for us what we should be doing for ourselves. He does not exempt us from problems, nor does he treat us like infants when we should be mature in our faith.

"Consider it pure joy, my brothers, whenever you face trials of many kinds, because you know that the testing of your faith develops perseverance. Perseverance must finish its work so that you may be mature and complete, not lacking anything" (James 1:2-4).

SUBTLE CHANGES

W hen we look back, we realize that Joan's illness must have begun about three years ago. We thought she'd retired early to enjoy life and to get away from the pressures of having to learn all about the computerization craze. What we didn't know at the time was that simple calculations had become major obstacles for her to work through. Our personal bills at home became delinquent due to her forgetfulness. Appointments with her clients became over-scheduled or broken. She knew all along something was terribly wrong.

Practical Suggestions

Changes associated with Alzheimer's Disease are said to be insidious — meaning that they don't appear to be as serious initially as they eventually turn out. Compounding the difficulty with identification and diagnosis is the person's ability to cover up his or her mistakes.

It is only after the disease has been allowed to run its course that the individual can no longer hide these mistakes, bringing to the attention of the family that there is a serious problem. Usually a full-blown crisis brings about the need to have the individual seen by a medical professional.

Families are strongly encouraged to seek medical assistance in order to obtain a proper diagnosis. Many different illnesses mimic and appear to be similiar to Alzheimer's Disease. These other diseases may cause permanent damage if allowed to run their courses without medical intervention.

It is essential that your loved one have a complete medical, neurological and psychiatric evaluation. Contact your local Alzheimer's Association for names of physicians that specialize in geriatric medicine and have a special interest in this disease.

Devotional

"Hindsight is 20-20." We can look back on the past and put the pieces of the puzzle together so much better than we could when we were living through the experiences.

Sometimes this hindsight makes us feel foolish: "Why didn't I sense at the time that something was wrong?"

Sometimes we feel angry at others. "The doctor should have known there was a serious problem!"

At other times hindsight makes us regretful: "I should have been more sympathetic through those early symptoms. I wish I would have taken advantage of the opportunity to communicate while there was still time."

There is some value in understanding the past. A clearer understanding of what has transpired in the past gives us an advantage in facing the reality of the present. But there is greater value in focusing on the future. When driving a car, an occasional glance in the rear view mirror is helpful, but your primary attention should be on the road ahead.

Clebe McClary barely escaped death in the Vietnam war. But he was maimed for life. He lost an arm and an eye and received a permanent injury to his leg. If anyone has a right to be bitter about the past, Clebe McClary does.

Yet this permanently disabled veteran has a vibrant, joyful and infectious personality. He speaks to thousands across America and inspires them to live each day to the fullest. His motto for life is this: "F-I-D-O." In fact those letters are on the license plate of his car. The letters stand for "Forget It and Drive On!"

Don't spend the rest of your days trying to reconstruct how the events of the past gradually unfolded. You will never understand those events fully, and there comes a time to "forget it and drive on."

"Brothers, I do not consider myself yet to have taken hold of it. But one thing I do: Forgetting what is behind and straining toward what is ahead, I press on toward the goal to win the prize for which God has called me heavenward in Christ Jesus" (Philippians 3:13-14).

CUING
(PROMPTING)

T he social worker at the hospital suggested that we use prompts such as small signs to help Jill find her way through our house. "Cuing," as she called it, will help orient and direct my wife with finding household items more easily.

Our granddaughter chuckled at the sight of our home being pasted with cartoon-like pictures everywhere. A picture of a toilet here, a kitchen appliance there. How sad to think that without these markers, Jill would be hopelessly lost within a home that she designed and lived in for some thirty years.

Practical Suggestions

In the early stages of Alzheimer's Disease the individual has difficulty with short term memory. Remote memory about events that took place years ago is usually still intact. They may be able to clearly remember facts about issues that happened twenty years ago but cannot remember what they did just a short time ago.

This keen sense of recall about one's earlier experience is often puzzling to caregivers since they have difficulty understanding why persons struggle with their daily activities. As the disease progresses, both recent and remote memory become impaired.

Cuing or prompting provides memory impaired individuals with visual pictures that may improve their ability to recognize and locate areas or items within their environments. Signs, with graphic illustrations identifying specific household rooms or utensils, allow individuals to recognize and associate with their intended activity or use. If you place familiar landmarks such as pictures or color guides at designated areas, the individual is guided by a directional road map.

The caregiver should attempt to maintain consistency in the environment, making special efforts not to rearrange furnishings. Tasks such as dressing and eating are more easily accomplished by laying out the items in sequential order. This activity reduces the need for the individual to make difficult decisions.

Let them maintain as much independence in their decision making as possible. If an activity requires a lot of complex decision making, which is unsettling to the person, then choices should be limited.

Devotional

Children may giggle when they see strange signs in your home. Try not to be offended. In fact, maybe laughter is a good response for you, too. It is possible to laugh at the humor in a situation without laughing at the person who is ill. Solomon said, "A cheerful heart is good medicine, but a crushed spirit dries up the bones" (Proverbs 17:22). Laughter helps to release tension, unite people and remind us that there is still hope. "Weeping may remain for a night, but rejoicing comes in the morning" (Psalm 30:5).

Nobody suffered more than Job. He lost all of his possessions, his ten children were killed tragically in a storm, and then his health began to fail him. Yet in the midst of his troubles he was reminded, "[God] will yet fill your mouth with laughter and your lips with shouts of joy" (Job 8: 21).

Laughter is not sacrilegious or disrespectful. Sometimes it is the best medicine for a heavy heart.

ECHOLALIA
(SPEECH)

D uring the past several weeks, I've noticed a gradual change in Tom's speech. He has begun to pick up phrases that he hears and repeats them continuously. It reminds me of our old Victrola stuck on the record. When I asked him why he does this, he just stares at me as if nothing had happened.

Practical Suggestions

Echolalia is exhibited through the repetition and imitation of speech or words heard. Caregivers should explore the possibility that the individual may be seeking reassurance and a sense of security.

When the individual exhibits this type of behavior, the caregiver should assess whether there is any particular pattern or trend taking place. Ask yourself what has happened recently in the environment that might have caused this behavior. Has a daily schedule been changed? Are visitors such as small children upsetting the individual?

When communicating with the person, it is important to make good eye contact with the individual and use short, simple words. Reply in a caring and responsive way and avoid confrontation or arguing with the individual as this may intensify his or her behavior. Use both verbal and nonverbal means of communication and, if necessary, write down statements for those who can still read.

Diversion is usually a good method to distract the individual as you may want to change the subject completely or engage him or her in some other activity.

Devotional

Though you cannot control the speech of others, you can make sure to control your own tongue. "He who loves a pure heart and whose speech is gracious will have the king for his friend" (Proverbs 22:11).

Booker T. Washington was the founder and president of Tuskeegee Institute, the first black college in Alabama. Once when he was walking to the school, an elderly woman called out to him, "Come here, boy, and chop some wood for me." Without a word of protest, the college president took off his coat, chopped the wood and carried it inside the woman's house.

When the woman discovered Washington's status, she was embarrassed and went to his office to apologize. "I'm so sorry," she said. "I didn't know who you were."

"That's all right," Washington replied. "I'm always eager to do a favor for a friend."

It is said that the woman became one of Tuskeegee Institute's most generous supporters.

It is easy to be kind to those who show you kindness. The true test occurs when the person will not, or cannot, reciprocate. God's love is evident in us when we are gracious to those who may not always be gracious to us.

"Let your conversation be always full of grace, seasoned with salt, so that you may know how to answer everyone" (Colossians 4:6).

SELF - PITY

This disease has really taken its toll on me. I often wonder about all of the plans we had after retirement. I feel so cheated, so unable to get my mind focused clearly.

Today, it finally dawned on me. Here I am feeling sorry for myself and I can't help but think how he must feel. Not being able to communicate or to take control, how frightening that must be.

Practical Suggestions

One of the most difficult issues that I have discovered through discussions with caregiver families over the years is the progressive stages of this disease. Categorically, we define the symptoms of Alzheimer's Disease as falling into three stages: early, middle, and late or final.

Unfortunately, the symptoms and behaviors of these stages are interchangeable and no two people demonstrate the exact progression of these behaviors according to the textbooks. Caring for someone with Alzheimer's Disease is not a concrete science; it has no set of instructional guides where you can follow certain procedures.

Caregiving affects longstanding relationships between two individuals. Feelings of self-pity, doubt, anger and even resentment are quite common. The caregiver may often feel a strong sense of being robbed or cheated of his or her marriage. This "Why me?" attitude can have devastating effects on the caregiver if not addressed appropriately.

Though being a caregiver may drastically change one's role as a marriage partner, it also provides a unique set of challenges that can be personally rewarding. Mastering new responsibilities can provide the caregiver with a stronger sense of self-esteem and self-worth.

Recognizing one's feelings through verbalization and accepting the inability to change what has already taken place allow him or her to move ahead in the role of caregiver.

Devotional

Ray and Ethel had been married for almost 50 years when Ray began having to take care of Ethel. When Ray could no longer care for Ethel at home, he carefully selected a nursing home within one mile of their home. For nearly two years Ray visited three times a day, helping to feed, bathe and give Ethel her medicine.

At Ethel's funeral, someone commended Ray for being so faithful to his wife through those last few difficult years. Ray said, "Well, you know, I made a promise to her 47 years ago to be faithful 'In sickness and in health.'"

Instead of feeling sorry for himself, Ray focused on doing what was right. To him, it was simply keeping a promise. Though his wife could not respond, Ray continued to do his duty. It was his way of thanking Ethel for the years of companionship and happiness she had given him.

Paul wrote, "Do nothing out of selfish ambition or vain conceit, but in humility consider others better than yourselves" (Philippians 2:3).

The surest way to unhappiness is to focus on yourself — what you don't have, how life has cheated you, the problems you face. But a sure way to fulfillment in life is to forget yourself and seek to serve others.

LOVE

Through all of our years of marriage, nothing has been more testing and challenging than the struggle with this disease. My thoughts take me back to our earlier days of parenting, buying our first home, and preparing our kids for college. These events now seem so trivial compared to this situation.

With each passing day and the responsibilities of caregiving, our relationship changes. Our love for each other is now shown in a different manner — new roles, new responsibilities. This illness is just another test of our lasting commitment to each other.

Practical Suggestions

As Alzheimer's Disease progresses, the love between the caregiver and the individual afflicted is tested daily. Adjustments to the relationship must be made to compensate for the changing roles of each partner.

Caregivers are often faced with new challenges and responsibilities that are drastically different from their previous roles. It is important that caregivers redefine their personal expectations in their new roles. One's expectations should be flexible, allowing for ongoing changes in the individual's behavior and abilities.

Spouses should recognize and address their own limitations and personal needs. Identify areas of responsibilities that you feel inadequate or uncomfortable in addressing. Finances, for example, may have always been handled by the afflicted spouse. The caregiver should seek assistance with this activity through someone knowledgeable in this subject. Attempt to break these areas down into small action plans.

Remember to set realistic and measurable goals which will

allow you to identify accomplished outcomes. Solicit input from family members or other caregivers who may be able to provide you with additional insight.

Devotional

Many people regard love as an involuntary emotion. They mistakenly think love is something you can fall into like falling into a ditch. They also think you can fall out of love like falling out of a tree.

But real love is much deeper than an emotion. It is an act of the will. You **decide** to love someone and to put that person's needs above your own.

I Corinthians 13, often called the "love chapter" of the Bible, says nothing about how you should feel when you love someone. But it says a lot about how love behaves: "Love is patient, love is kind . . . love does not keep a record of wrongs . . . love never fails."

Feelings will fail and emotions will fluctuate. W.A. Criswell had been married to his wife for fifty years when he said, "Sometimes I love my wife so much I could just eat her up. Then the next day I wish I had!"

Shallow people base their love on how they feel at the time. But authentic love does the right thing for the other person regardless of emotions. Romance will fade away, but true love never fails.

MISUNDERSTANDING

H ad we really explained to our grandchildren what was wrong with their Grandpa? This past Thanksgiving, we were so overprotective of Jack's illness that we shut the grandchildren off from him.

They must have wondered, what had they done? Why couldn't they play with Grandpa as they did in the past? His illness has taken away one of the most cherished moments of our lives, that of being a grandparent.

Practical Suggestions

We tend to think that Alzheimer's Disease affects only the elderly. Unfortunately, we realize that this disease affects the entire family. Children often conceptualize illness with bandages or being confined in bed. How confusing it must be to explain to them that Grandpa is sick. On the outside he appears to be perfectly normal; on the inside, however, his mind is slowly slipping away.

A child's encounter with a family member having Alzheimer's Disease can all too often be negative unless he or she has some understanding of the disease. It is important to explain and properly discuss the disease and behaviors with children.

Caregivers should plan accordingly for family visits. During the holidays, be careful not to overload the individual with too much change in his or her daily routines. Stimulus overload can cause increased restlessness, pacing and even agitation.

If necessary, decrease the amount of visitation time and keep child-oriented activities to a minimum. Remove the person from the immediate surroundings when activities appear to be upsetting to them.

Devotional

The task of being a grandparent is much deeper than "doting" over the grandchildren or spoiling them. Children often learn about the realities of life and the aging process from observing their grandparents. Children need to learn that life is not always comfortable and easy. Those who are protected from the reality of illness are not prepared for real life. Jesus said,"In this world you will have trouble" (John 16:33).

As grandparents you have the opportunity to teach your grandchildren several valuable lessons about life. When children see one of their grandparents struggling with a disease and the other lovingly caring for the one who is ill, it will deepen their understanding of love, commitment, aging and suffering.

You also have the opportunity to teach them that it is possible to be joyful in the midst of suffering. When they see you enduring trials without losing your ability to laugh and be kind to others, then they learn that suffering is not an excuse for bitterness or a hard heart.

"Teach the older women to be reverent in the way they live . . . to teach what is good. Then they can train the younger women to love their husbands and children" (Titus 2:3-4). Demonstrate for your grandchildren what it means "to love and to cherish till death do us part."

AWARENESS

I painstakingly listened to the conversation that Mary had with our good friends, the Williams. Her jumbled words and inability to stay focused really brought to my attention how "out of it" she has become. It's difficult for me to see and accept how this disease has affected her, affected us. I can no longer allow myself to deny and rationalize the destruction that this disease has brought into our lives. The reality of its devastation becomes more apparent with each passing day.

Practical Suggestions

Aphasia is the inability to properly communicate or express oneself through speech. As Alzheimer's Disease progresses, the individual's ability to express oneself becomes more impaired.

Problems with speech may include difficulty in recalling words, jumbling, paraphrasing, using inappropriate comments and difficulty in making a point. This rambling-on response becomes obvious to the caregiver as the individual's ability to communicate declines.

Factors that enhance communication include providing the individual with an environment that is non-rushed. Distractions such as noise, or numerous visual movements in the immediate area, can be overwhelming to the person.

Encourage the individual to take his or her time and speak in slow, short phrases. Be sure to allow plenty of response time and try not to interrupt his or her reply with additional questions or statements. Ask questions that require yes or no answers rather than complex discussions.

Devotional

When our loved ones make mistakes around others, we are sometimes embarrassed for them — and for ourselves. We may even be afraid our friends will no longer want us around, or that they might be losing respect for us.

A wise older friend once advised me: "Don't apologize for your kids. If people have had children, they understand. If they don't have children, no amount of explaining will enable them to understand!"

The same is true with Alzheimer's Disease. Those who understand the situation will be supportive, while those who are ignorant about the problem may not change their attitudes even with a detailed explanation.

Someone said, "If you worry too much about what others think of you, then you would probably be disappointed to discover how seldom they did." Don't be overly concerned about the reaction of others. Good friends will be supportive.

"A friend loves at all times,
and a brother is born
for adversity"

(Proverbs 17:17).

RUSHING

One thing is for certain with this disease, the responsibilities of caregiving never end. Where in the world does the time go? I find it nearly impossible to get all the things done that I want to do each day.

This endless pace of giving and giving is beginning to wear on me. I've learned to balance those things that must get done and leave those that are not so important for another day.

I keep telling myself that physical and emotional rest are essential if I'm to maintain this pace. If I can't take care of myself, how will I ever be able to care for my husband?

Practical Suggestions

Caregiving requires the balance of providing the necessary assistance and yet not overextending oneself to the point of burnout. In our mad rush to get everything done, we must be careful not to overdo it.

It is important that caregivers take a well-needed time out from the day-to-day activities of providing for their loved ones. Alzheimer's Disease is said to have two victims, the individual afflicted with the disease and the caregiver. I once worked with a caregiver who was so determined to take care of every need of her husband that she finally exhausted herself to the point of requiring hospitalization. Fortunately, she had the necessary family resources to care for her husband while she recuperated.

Caregiver burnout is usually facilitated by the caregiver's withdrawing from his or her social contacts and becoming isolated. It can lead to physical symptoms including high blood pressure, nervous disorders and even heart disease.

As the disease progresses and the responsibilities increase, isolation can create an overwhelming environment for the caregiver. Isolation compounded with little affirmation and appreciation for one's increased efforts can severely put the caregiver at risk for physical and emotional problems.

Explore alternative options to assist you with some of your daily routines. Actively engage other family members or friends in assisting and providing you with some well-deserved respite. In our haste to constantly push and drive ourselves, we must realize that eventually this drive leads to an empty gas tank! Take time and refuel.

Devotional

Everyone has limits. Anyone involved in caregiving needs to take an occasional break from the demands.

A woman in need of healing once made her way through the crowd and touched the hem of Jesus' garment. She was immediately healed, but Jesus turned around and said, "Who touched me?"

Those standing nearby reminded Him that anyone in the crowd could have bumped into Him. But the Bible says that Jesus knew power had gone out from Him. He turned to say something comforting to the woman He had just healed. Healing others drained Jesus of power and energy.

That is why Jesus needed times of rest and renewal. He occasionally hiked up a mountain where he spent the day alone, away from people, resting and praying. He would sometimes get into a friend's boat and ask to be taken to the other side of the lake to escape the demanding crowds and daily pressures for a while.

A preacher boasted, "I never take a vacation, because the devil never does!"

One of his exasperated church members mumbled, "That's one of the many ways he resembles the devil."

If Jesus Christ needed times of renewal, how much more do we! If you want to have the power and love needed to be a healer and caregiver, take time away. You need it, and your loved one needs you at your best.

CONTROL

I say to myself over and over again, "I've got to get control of my emotions and feelings." I can't let this disease destroy me, too. Control is so crucial to my own survival and sanity — not knowing what to expect, what hurdles lie ahead. I know I can and must overcome them, no matter how difficult they seem. Being in control, I have the confidence to take each day one step at a time. With each success I realize I CAN do it!

Practical Suggestions

Control is often defined as the ability to influence the actions and behavior of others. It is difficult at best for caregivers to predict the behavior of their loved ones with Alzheimer's Disease.

Caregivers should attempt to be flexible in their desires to meet set goals. Rigidity with control issues can lead to disappointment and frustration.

Control over day-to-day activities is enhanced greatly through knowledge of the disease. An example is the limited amount of time caregivers have to do things such as shopping while still providing supervision for their loved one. Respite care services may provide you with the necessary free time to carry out these tasks. Awareness and the utilization of local resources allows you to develop alternative strategies in dealing with difficult situations.

Caregivers have better control over unpredictable situations when they feel in control. This self-assurance is often developed through the experience and knowledge of the clinical manifestations of the disease.

Once you know what you're dealing with, it's a lot easier to develop a game plan. Don't forget to develop a regular routine for exercise and be sure this program includes a nourishing diet.

Devotional

There are some situations that you can and should control. Have you ever lain in bed in the middle of the night, fuming because the house is cold, instead of getting up to get the extra blanket in the closet ten feet away? It is foolish to worry when you can and should control the situation yourself.

But there are other circumstances you cannot control. It is at those times that you must learn to be flexible and believe that God will provide the resources you need to cope with the challenge. It is during those times, when we know we cannot control things on our own, that we learn to trust in God.

I Corinthians 10:13 promises, "No temptation has seized you except what is common to man. And God is faithful; He will not let you be tempted beyond what you can bear. But when you are tempted, he will also provide a way out so that you can stand up under it."

I love the plaque that reads, "Lord, help me to understand that nothing will happen today that you and I can't handle together." Release to God those situations beyond your control.

SHAME

M y friends are sympathetic to my wife's illness. They express their feelings of shame. "It's a shame she can't talk. It's a shame she can't feed herself. It's a shame she doesn't know where she lives." Don't they realize that I don't need their shame? I need their support. I need them to get me through another day. That's the real shame.

Practical Suggestions

The unfortunate misunderstanding of Alzheimer's Disease and its effect on the individual can often elicit comments of pity and shame from friends and acquaintances. The old saying that "ignorance is bliss" comes to mind when I think about all of the comments people have made to caregivers.

It's a shame that they can't listen to their own comments. Sometimes I think that if they could, they would reconsider or think twice about what they say.

Occasional comments by friends may be distressing and upsetting to the caregiver. If given the opportunity, let others know how you are feeling. Don't allow feelings of anger to build up within you.

Individuals who are uncomfortable and unfamiliar with the effects of Alzheimer's Disease may be at odds about what they can do to be supportive. Turn a negative impression into a positive outcome. Caregivers should seek support and assistance from those individuals who can provide guidance.

Devotional

People sometimes say stupid things when they are trying to encourage us. I have a friend who often sings before large crowds. After one of her performances, a fan said to her, "You know, you look really pretty from a distance!"

71

When a friend makes a comment that hurts more than it helps, there are two ways you can respond. First, try to be understanding. Look beyond the words to the intentions. Your friend is probably trying to help and simply doesn't know what to say. He is probably trying to say, "I care about your situation."

The second response is to tactfully tell the truth about your feelings. Matthew 18:15 says, "If your brother sins against you, go and show him his fault, just between the two of you. If he listens to you, you have won your brother over."

You could tactfully say, "You are right — it is a shame she can't feed herself. But it would help me if you would encourage me instead of pitying us. I am weak, and I need you as a friend to strengthen me because you mean a great deal to me."

Your comment may hurt your friend a little, but a true friendship will benefit from such tactful honesty. "Wounds from a friend can be trusted, but an enemy multiplies kisses" (Proverbs 27:6).

ACHIEVEMENT

Today, I was very proud of myself. I was not sure whether I was going to be able to complete this hectic schedule. I made it! Doctors' appointments, bank meetings, grocery shopping, dinner guests: the activities never seemed to end.

You know, when you stop and allow yourself to plan accordingly, these obstacles can be overcome. I sat and reflected about how far I've come as a caregiver. I've accomplished things that I never dreamed I could have mastered several months ago.

Practical Suggestions

Caregiver motivation is often achieved through the successful mastering of caregiver tasks and obstacles. Mastery over activities that once seemed impossible can boost the caregiver's self-esteem.

Achievement of caregiver activities is often enhanced through setting realistic goals for certain activities and breaking them down into small individualized steps. A male caregiver that I counseled was really distraught about his desire to maintain involvement with a civic organization whose annual meeting was out of town. He struggled with the need to care for his wife, yet he felt a strong need to maintain personal contact with this network. We discussed the possibility of gradually working toward an overnight trip. He arranged a sitter to care for his wife for extended periods of time. Finally, he was comfortable with leaving her overnight knowing that her needs would be met. His overnight visit went very smoothly and his wife handled his absence fine.

As a caregiver, it is important to break down tasks into small steps. Once you successfully have orchestrated smaller caregiver tasks you will begin to gain the confidence to take on larger responsibilities.

Repetition of certain caregiver activities allows one to master and fine tune these tasks over time. Remember, what may work for you today in handling certain situations may not be effective tomorrow. Acknowledge your achievement and do something special for yourself. You've earned it!

Devotional

A woodpecker was hammering at an oak tree during a thunderstorm when lightning struck his tree and split it in two. The stunned bird disappeared and returned later with five of his cronies. Nodding in the direction of the split oak tree he said, "Boys, I don't mean to brag, but my work is right over there!"

While you rejoice over what has been accomplished, remember to give God thanks for what he has done through you. Our achievements are "not by might, nor by power, but by My Spirit, say the Lord" (Zechariah 4:6).

You have prayed for help and God has given it. You are right to feel good about your work, but remember to give thanks to the One who is "the giver of every good and perfect gift" (James 1:17).

Commit to memory Philippians 4:13, and repeat it several times today: "I can do everything through Him who gives me strength."

ATTITUDE

A lzheimer's Disease was not a choice in our lives that we opted to have; it just happened. How I deal with its aftermath, however, is a choice that I can make. I guess I could feel sorry for myself, be a martyr, but life still goes on. This disease has given me the realization that life does go on and I can either be miserable or give it my best shot. Life is still very precious, no matter what we've been dealt.

Practical Suggestions

Undoubtedly, Alzheimer's Disease places many restrictions on the individual and on the caregiver. However, the freedom and control to choose and decide which course of treatment to pursue still lies with the caregiver.

Personal attitudes regarding your role as caregiver weigh heavily in how successful you will be over the long haul of this disease. Caregiver success is often measured by one's ability to perform daily hands-on responsibilities and not to fall victim to the rigorous demands of caregiving.

Learn as much as possible about this disease and get "connected" with a support group early in the disease process. Finally, take care of your own spiritual, physical, and emotional needs.

Devotional

Jeff Keith lost a leg to cancer when he was a child. But in 1985, at the age of 22, Jeff spent eight months running more than 3,000 miles across the United States. He wore out 35 pairs of running shoes, and his artificial leg was replaced five times as he maintained a pace of twelve miles a day! When Jeff had finished, not only had he raised over $120,000 for the American Cancer Society, he had also raised the consciousness of people about those with disabilities. He said, "I wanted to show that people like me are physically challenged, not physically handicapped."

The difference between Jeff Keith and a healthy young person who wallows in self-pity is not circumstances, but attitude. You have been dealt a set of challenging circumstances. But remember what one man said: "Suffering is inevitable in this world; misery is optional." Joy is possible even in the midst of suffering. The difference is attitude.

No one suffered more — physically and emotionally — than Jesus Christ. Yet His disciples were attracted to Him because of His joy, peace and hope.

"Your attitude should be the same as that of Christ Jesus" (Philippians 2:5).

REMINISCING
(RECALL)

*I*t's hard to believe that a disease as devastating as Alzheimer's allows my wife to remember exact details about events that happened years ago. Her keen sense of detail about specific activities from our past is remarkable. Yet, she has great difficulty remembering what she did this morning or even moments earlier. Reminiscing and talking about the past bring out a kind of realness in her, a state of control and surety about herself that isn't there otherwise.

Practical Suggestions

During the early stages of Alzheimer's Disease, the individual's ability to recall recent events is impaired. Remote memory is still very much intact, allowing the individual to discuss in specific detail events that happened many years ago.

As the disease progresses, the individual's ability to recall previous events may become more difficult. Since defense mechanisms are still very much intact in the early stages of the illness, many months or years may pass before one can no longer cover up his or her mistakes.

Caregivers should use concrete information and examples that differentiate the "here and now" from the past. It is important to note that the individual with Alzheimer's Disease can mask, or cover up their inabilities, reducing the awareness of potential problems.

Caregivers should be both supportive and patient when trying to clarify historical facts. Be careful not to become argumentative over specific details. Reminiscing therapy can often have a calming effect on an individual who is restless or upset. This technique attempts to elicit pleasant memories from the person's earlier life through the use of familiar pictures, music or other personal items.

I once worked with a woman in a nursing home who wouldn't respond to any verbal communication. After months of unsuccessful attempts by staff to get her to speak and share her feelings she was taken to a music therapy session. After hearing several old-time gospel songs, the woman began to join and sing along. She finally opened up and began to speak.

Explore the use of these types of activities with your loved one. Carefully assess the materials used, as some events in their past lives may be upsetting.

Devotional

As you have discovered, memory is a tremendous blessing that we often take for granted. But it can also be a curse. Guilt, resentment, insecurity and low self-esteem are difficult to over-come because we have such good memories.

There are blessings even in the greatest tragedies. It is a horrible thing to lose your memory, but there are times when it could be a Godsend. People suffering from emotional trauma are sometimes given shock treatments to block the unpleasant experiences from their minds.

God promises that in heaven we won't be able to recall those events that brought us pain and suffering. "Behold, I will create new heavens and a new earth. The former things will not be remembered, nor will they come to mind" (Isaiah 65:17).

One of the amazing characteristics of God is his ability to forget our sins. He promises: "I am He who blots out your transgressions, for My own sake, and remembers your sins no more" (Isaiah 43:25).

Though it can be a tremendous burden to live with someone who is unable to recall the recent past, rejoice that some details of long ago are recalled. Share those pleasant memories with your loved one.

BATHING

Edgar refuses to bathe himself anymore. I keep on him about the fact that he's beginning to smell, yet he doesn't seem to care. He used to be so neat and clean. Now, he shaves once a week, if I'm lucky. He doesn't even want me to wash his clothes. This is one of my biggest battles as a caregiver —and one I seem to be losing.

Practical Suggestions

For the caregiver, bathing probably presents more of a challenge than any other activity of daily living. The unwillingness to bathe may be misinterpreted by the caregiver as stubbornness or lack of cooperation on the part of the individual.

However, bathing may bring a real sense of fear that is difficult for the loved one to overcome. Lack of coordination in the bathtub or shower may increase this fear, especially if the individual has fallen previously. To reduce this fear and anxiety the caregiver may want to try sponge baths as an alternative.

The gradual decline of the individual's senses poses potential risk, due to water temperature (burns) as well as falls. Other helpful tips when assisting with bathing include explaining prior to each action what will be done and the reason for it. Provide a consistent routine and schedule based on previous patterns. When approaching the individual in the bathroom, be sure to use slow direct movements. Do not rush or surprise the person.

If the person is going to take a bath, have the water ready prior to the person going into the bathroom. The sound of running water and the "echo" effect of conversations may be frightening to them.

When the individual is in the bath, look for any aspects of bathing that might be upsetting or that might trigger fear. Use careful movements while assisting the person with bathing and be sensitive to the possible risks associated with this activity.

Safety bars and supports in the bathtub can help reduce the potential risk of falls. Always provide the person with positive reinforcement for his or her personal accomplishments.

Devotional

On the night before his death, Jesus washed the feet of his disciples. The Son of God, stooping to wash the smelly, dirty feet of fishermen and tax collectors, provided a dramatic display of humility and service.

But Simon Peter protested. "Lord," he said, "you will never wash my feet." Perhaps Peter objected because he was humiliated by his own failure to wash Jesus' feet when He first entered. Maybe Peter just felt awkward. He must have felt very uncomfortable when the One in authority over him began washing his feet.

But Jesus said, "Peter, if I don't wash your feet, you have no part in me."

"Then wash my head and hands as well as my feet," Peter said. Peter was one of those people who took everything to extremes.

But Jesus said, "You are already clean. You don't need a bath. But just as I your Lord and Master wash your feet, so you are to wash the feet of one another." Jesus was not speaking literally of washing others' feet. Foot-washing was an act of service, and Jesus wanted them to learn to serve one another.

Jesus said, "Whoever wants to become great among you must be your servant." You will never be more like Jesus than when you stoop to help another. Those you serve may not fully appreciate your sacrifice — they may even protest against it. But the Lord appreciates your act of caring. He promised that even a cup of cold water given in His name would have its reward.

DRIVING

L ast night Bill walked in the door as if something serious had happened. He was gone almost two hours longer than usual. I knew something was wrong. He looked bewildered and upset. Finally, he told me that he had been driving around frantically looking for our house. Nothing appeared to be familiar to him as he aimlessly rode around our neighborhood.

Practical Suggestions

Few issues play more havoc on the caregiver than having to address the issue of driver safety. Losing one's driving privileges denies the individual the freedom and control to come and go as he or she pleases and has been accustomed to for many years.

It is essential that caregivers limit, and eliminate if necessary, the person's opportunity to drive when their ability and judgment to handle the operation of a vehicle is impaired. Driving skills required to adequately handle a vehicle include perception, cognition and execution of motor skills.

Unfortunately, as Alzheimer's Disease progresses all three of these areas are affected. Caregivers should assess the severity of the individual's impairment and intervene accordingly when necessary.

Assess the person's driving environment and make modifications if needed. For example, a driver can be limited to shorter trips or only driving during the daytime. Consideration should be given to the geographical location of your residence. Obviously, rural traffic and roadways will differ significantly from the city and its superhighways.

When it is necessary to restrict or eliminate driving privileges, you can solicit the help and assistance of authority figures. Family physicians and/or attorneys may be able to convince the person that it is time to give up his or her driving privilege.

When all else fails, disable the vehicle so it is unusable. Loss of this privilege can often have emotional and psychological effects on the person. Through the proper planning and coordination of alternative transportation means, some of these effects can be avoided.

Devotional

We've all heard the advertisement slogan: "Friends don't let friends drive drunk." Someone who lets an intoxicated friend get into a car and drive off is showing cowardice, not friendship. It is in the best interest of the one you love and of others who will meet him on the road for you to intervene. You don't want him to feel insulted, but the wise and loving thing for you to do is to insist that he does not drive.

The Bible says, "Which of you, if his son . . . asks for a fish, will give him a snake? If you, then, though you are evil, know how to give good gifts to your children, how much more will your Father in heaven give good gifts to those who ask Him!" (Matthew 7:11). A wise, generous father responds affirmatively to positive requests of his children.

But the wise father also says "no" to requests that are potentially harmful. If the son asked for a snake, most parents would say "No way!" In the same way, if a six-year-old asked for a gun, or a twelve-year-old wanted to start dating, or a fourteen-year-old wanted a motorcycle, a loving parent would say "no." The child maybe disappointed, but your inacquiescence is in the best interest of the child and of everyone else concerned.

When we love someone who has limited mental capacity, sometimes the most loving and courageous thing we can do is to refuse to honor a request. Your loved one may be disappointed or irritated, but remember that "love always protects" (I Corinthians 13:7).

COPING

Through thick and thin I've somehow been able to adjust to all of Lynn's needs. As I look back, I find it hard to believe that I've made it this far. Did I do all of the right things? Probably not. I did them the best way I knew how. It wasn't always easy and it surely wasn't always pleasant.

Practical Suggestions

Coping mechanisms are ways that caregivers use in adjusting to caregiving demands without forfeiting their overall goals and objectives. As caregivers, we constantly develop new coping strategies through an ongoing process of trial and error.

We sharpen our caregiver skills through the use of educational materials. Participation in support groups, where we are exposed to helpful tips from seasoned caregivers, is also a way to improve coping skills.

There are many successful ways to handle specific patient behaviors. No simple response works for everyone all of the time. Adaptability and flexibility to meet these challenges are probably the most important characteristic traits of a caregiver. The ability to perceive and anticipate a patient's needs is crucial for coping and is the hallmark of a good caregiver.

Devotional

A child may have a difficult time noticing very much physical growth if he measures himself against the doorpost every week. In the same way, we usually don't see the spiritual maturity that is gradually taking place in us. In fact, those times when we think we are only coping may be the times we are experiencing the most spiritual growth.

"Consider it pure joy, my brothers, whenever you face trials of many kinds, because you know that the testing of your faith develops perseverance. Perseverance must finish its work so that you may be mature and complete, not lacking anything" (James 1:2-4).

Adversity can make you bitter or it can make you better. The same sun that melts butter hardens clay. The fact that you have persevered to this point is evidence that you are allowing God to develop your character and deepen your faith. You are passing the test. Congratulations!

MOURNING

My husband's condition has worsened significantly these past couple of weeks. I've really felt a change come over me that I don't know how to explain. Our family doctor says that I'm going through anticipatory grief or mourning. He says that I'm preparing myself for the inevitable. One moment I find myself trying to rationalize that things will be O.K., and the next I'm angry and resentful for what this disease has put us through these past several years.

Practical Suggestions

After many years of providing for their loved ones, caregivers have faced many losses, but none so final as that of death. Anticipatory mourning is a defense mechanism often exhibited by caregivers in various stages of caring for an Alzheimer's patient. Individuals may experience an emotional roller coaster: feeling angry one moment and being at a total loss the next. This grieving process is a normal reaction and fosters a process of healing and working through the associated stress and pain.

It is not uncommon for the caregiver to experience both physical and psychological symptoms. As the patient evolves through the various stages of the disease, you and your family will be faced with many difficult decisions. Discuss advanced directives with other family members. Also evaluate the resources necessary to formalize your final plans. As difficult as it may seem at the time, you should consider an autopsy to confirm the diagnosis and to provide much-needed research data. Making arrangements for the autopsy before your loved one dies will facilitate the process at the time of death. Your local chapter of the Alzheimer's Association can provide information about autopsy arrangements in your state.

Devotional

One of my favorite authors is the late Bob Benson. He had a homespun way of making the profound simple and making hope come alive. Bob was a gregarious, people-loving person. When he wrote his last book, he knew he was dying of cancer. In his book he said that he used to think of dying as "leaving the party early." But facing death made him realize that, in reality, there was a party going on somewhere else, and "I'm missing out on it," he said.

The Bible calls that party "the marriage supper of the Lamb," where we will "sit down with Abraham, Isaac and Jacob in the Kingdom." If we will sit down with those patriarchs in heaven, we can be assured we will be sitting with Christians of our day, too.

I especially like the title of Bob Benson's final book: *See You at the House.* If you are a part of a large, loving family, then the phrase "see you back at the house" communicates that you are soon going to be reunited at a place where there is love, laughter, acceptance, security and fellowship.

Jesus said, "In my Father's house are many rooms; if it was not so, I would have told you. I am going there to prepare a place for you" (John 14:2).

We can say to those who have died, and to those who are dying, "I'll see you one day at the Father's house."

PARANOIA

Today, my wife became enraged because she felt someone had stolen her sweater. She continues to think that there is a plot to get her and that our children and I are scheming against her. I had to stop her the other day from calling the police. She was sure that some stranger had broken into our home and had gone through all of her drawers. I found her sweater later sitting in our microwave.

Practical Suggestions

It is quite common for individuals with Alzheimer's Disease to forget where they have placed personal items. As the disease progresses, the individual may become less aware of his or her own actions.

As reasoning capabilities diminish, the person may become suspicious and paranoid. Paranoid ideation is perhaps the most distressing behavior for the burdened family. Not only are the caregiver's efforts going unrecognized and unappreciated, but patients truly may believe that the family is abusing them and is scheming to take advantage of their misfortunes. One of the common characteristics of paranoia is mistrust.

People with paranoid personalities are constantly on their guard because they see their immediate surroundings as a threatening and unsafe place. The surrounding events and actions may be misconstrued as plots to "get" the person. The individual may be expressing signs of fear and anxiety and the caregiver should provide support and reassurance.

Be careful not to engage in a confrontation or argument as this may only make matters worse. Usually, a search of the premises turns up the misplaced items and provides the individual with a sense of security. It may be necessary to seek medical attention if the person's behavior becomes unmanageable.

Devotional

We are born with only two innate fears: the fear of falling, and the fear of loud noises. All other fears are learned, and most of them come from the enemy of man's soul.

However, some fear is helpful and necessary. Children should fear traffic in a busy street. Teens should fear diseases that can be contracted sexually. Adults should fear imprisonment. Jesus told us to fear the One who had the power to destroy our body and soul in hell. Sometimes fear motivates us to appropriate behavior.

But unfounded fear destroys happiness and peace of mind and makes others apprehensive. While you cannot alleviate all the fears in the mind of your loved one, you can refuse to allow fear to dominate your own life.

"So we say with confidence, 'The Lord is my helper; I will not be afraid. What can man do to me?' " (Hebrews 13:6).

TRUST

I no longer explain all the facts to my husband. He can't handle all the details and it seems to only upset him. Sometimes, I feel bad that I'm withholding information from him. We've always based our relationship on honest and open communication. I find myself trying to make up things because he gets so confused and upset. When I do explain things, he gets them so messed up. Today, I made some changes with our financial investments. I wouldn't have dared to think of making these changes without his knowledge prior to his illness. Now he has no idea what I'm doing.

Practical Suggestions

Caregivers are often faced with the dilemma as to how much information and details they should share with their loved ones. Withholding information can instill a sense of disloyalty and guilt in the caregiver. As a general rule of thumb, the caregiver should provide as much information as the person is capable of handling. When you find it difficult for the person to understand or tolerate information, simply back off.

It is important to keep in perspective that the individual's ability to comprehend becomes impaired over time due to the disease process. Communication techniques need to be readjusted based on the individual's ability to understand and interpret messages. Provide small pieces of information at a time. Complex conversations requiring the individual to process a lot of information may be too much for the person to handle. When in doubt, remember to keep your messages simple.

Devotional

Jesus recognized the limitations of His disciples and withheld some information from them. "I have much more to say to you, more than you can now bear" (John 16:12). It wasn't a lack of trust that motivated Jesus to limit what He told His followers. He just recognized that they could only absorb and comprehend so much at that time. His response was loving, and so is yours.

While you deeply regret that your mate is not capable of assimilating all the facts, do not feel guilty about withholding some information. You are not being dishonest, nor are you displaying a lack of trust. You are acknowledging the reality of his limitations and accepting the responsibility that has been placed upon your shoulders. You are making decisions that must be made and you are responding in love. "Love always protects" (I Corinthians 13:7).

Corrie ten Boom was one of the great saints of this century. Prior to her arrest by the Nazis and her confinement in a concentration camp, Corrie had helped her family hide runaway Jews in their home in Holland. If a member of the Gestapo knocked on the door of the Boom house while they were hiding a Jewish family and asked, "Are you harboring a Jew in this house?" a completely honest answer would have been "yes." But sharing all the information would not have been the wise or loving thing to do. The Hebrew midwives in the Old Testament are honored for taking such action and saving the lives of the Hebrew babies out of the hand of Pharaoh.

Without question, it is sometimes necessary to conceal some of the facts. We must pray that God would give us the wisdom necessary to determine when to explain all the facts and when to keep silent.

FALLS

In my attempt to create a safer home for Mary,
I may have created a bigger problem. I thought
that rearranging furniture would make it easier
for her to get around. Instead, she has fallen
several times in the past couple of days and
bruised herself pretty badly.

Practical Suggestions

An important element in providing a safe environment for
individuals with Alzheimer's Disease is maintaining familiarity and consistency in their surroundings. Changes such as
rearranging furniture can complicate matters and increase
confusion and disorientation.

There are many causes of falls and many of them easily
can be eliminated with little effort by the caregiver. First, it is
important to conduct an environmental assessment of your
residence. This should be done regularly as part of your overall fall prevention program. Search for various causes of falls
and correct them in a timely manner.

Consideration should be given to high risk areas, which
include bathrooms, stairways, family rooms and kitchens.
Caregivers should clearly mark steps and stairwell landings.
Keep all stairways and landings clear of any obstructions. Extension cords as well as telephone cords should be moved out
of passageways. If you use throw rugs in your home, be sure
that they are secured and replace their adhesive strips when
necessary.

Decline in the individual's functional abilities, particularly
his or her mobility, increases the potential for falls. Individuals who are unsteady on their feet should be supervised and
escorted when attempting to move about the room.

The physical environment can also be an important factor
in reducing falls. Attempt to create a living arrangement that
makes the best possible use of their vision. Eliminate the po-

tential for glare, enhance lighting and eliminate wall and floor coverings that blend. Handrails should be installed in appropriate areas to provide the individual with support and stability. Make sure that they are securely mounted to the walls.

Devotional

We all need stability and security in our lives. The world as we know it is rapidly changing. Computers, satellites, airplanes. nuclear power, fax machines and VCR's have created a culture vastly different from the one we knew 40 years ago.

Moral values that were considered absolute and unchanging 25 years ago are now being challenged and disregarded. In the play "Green Pastures" the angel reports to the Lord about the world's condition and says, "Everything nailed down is coming loose!" Don't you feel that way at times?

In addition to the cultural and moral changes our world is experiencing you are also experiencing the insecurity of a rapidly changing relationship. What once was steady and predictable has become shaky and unreliable. It takes all of your willpower not to fall, spiritually and emotionally.

In a world that is so unstable, rejoice that "Jesus Christ is the same yesterday, today, and forever" (Hebrews 13:8). He said, "Heaven and earth will pass away, but my words will never pass away" (Matthew 24:35).

We sing, "On Christ the solid rock I stand, all other ground is sinking sand."

Another hymn that expresses our prayer is this: "Change and decay in all around I see, O thou who changest not abide with me."

Trust today in the Lord's promise: "Cast your cares on the Lord and He will sustain you; He will never let the righteous fall" (Psalm 55:22).

SWALLOWING
(NOURISHMENT)

Roy doesn't seem to be able to keep any food down and has really lost interest in eating. When he does eat, he forgets to chew his food and often ends up choking. This afternoon at lunch he looked like a chipmunk hoarding food in his cheeks. He had totally forgotten that he had taken two big bites of food and had not swallowed.

Practical Suggestions

It is important for a caregiver to maintain the individual's highest level of functioning. Maintaining a well-balanced nutritional diet, as well as encouraging a regimented exercise program, is an essential component of providing care for the person with Alzheimer's Disease.

Daily cleanliness of the mouth and teeth is important in preventing infection and mouth sores. As the disease progresses individuals may exhibit a wide range of feeding difficulties including choking, spitting food, hoarding food in their cheeks, drooling, leaving their mouth open, biting or chewing on utensils and refusing to eat.

Caregivers can facilitate good nutritional intake through the substitution of finger foods and items that are easy to swallow. Limit the amount of food items the individual must choose from when eating. Significant weight loss should be discussed with your physician and supplemental nourishment may be necessary. Evaluate dentures to ensure proper fitting and assess for sharp edges that may be an irritant to the individual.

Devotional

You are to be commended for finding ways to feed your loved one physically when it is difficult to do. It's also important to continue feeding him/her spiritually. Jesus said, "man does not live on bread alone, but on every word that comes from the mouth of God" (Matthew 4:4).

I once visited a 39-year-old woman who was dying of cancer. She had been in a coma for over 24 hours and the doctors were predicting she would not live through the night. She had responded to no one that entire day.

I bent over her and identified myself, but she did not respond to me either. I squeezed her hand, but her hand remained limp. I said, "Donna, I want to pray with you."

In my prayer, I quoted Psalm 23, "The Lord is my shepherd, I shall not want." As I began the second line, I heard her whispering the Psalm with me: "He maketh me to lie down in green pastures . . ." Goose bumps broke out on my arms as she continued to repeat, "Yea, though I walk through the valley of the shadow of death, I will fear no evil, for thou art with me . . ."

When the prayer was completed, family members were standing around the bed weeping. She never whispered another word and died a few hours later. Donna did not respond to her family, her doctor or her minister, but she did respond to the truth of God's Word. In her hour of need, she was nourished and comforted.

Take time to read a brief Bible passage to your loved one every day. It may surprise you how much he is comforted, encouraged and fed by the meat and milk of God's Word. And you will be fed too.

AGGRESSION

M y son keeps on me to do something about John's aggressive behavior. This morning, without warning, he grabbed me by the arm and wanted to know who I was and why I was in his house. It frightened me at first, but then he settled down after I was able to convince him that I was his wife. He has these mood swings that are so unpredictable. I try not to let him know that he scares me.

Practical Suggestions

As Alzheimer's Disease progresses through its various stages, the individual may exhibit excessive mood swings, restlessness and agitation. This behavior, which we refer to as catastrophic reactions, may be triggered by excessive stimuli in the environment. Reactions such as these happen when the individual is overwhelmed by the immediate surroundings and cannot adequately respond to the situation.

The identification of causes is the first step that the caregiver should undertake in determining the appropriate management techniques. Caregivers may observe a degree of restlessness or agitation when daily routines are altered, posing increased activities around the person. Holidays, with increased visitation from family and friends, can be unsettling to the individual.

Developing caregiver strategies to manage this difficult behavior can be extremely challenging. Try to determine whether there is a relationship between the person's behavior and any possible changes in his or her environment. It may be beneficial to remove the individual from the upsetting stimuli and limit unnecessary activities. Remove potentially harmful items from the immediate surrounding that could pose dangers to yourself or to your loved one.

When appropriate, provide the person with opportunities to experience a sense of control. Attempts should be made to calm individuals and defuse their behavior through the use of nonverbal expression. When necessary, consult your family physician if this behavior intensifies or increases in frequency. Caution should be given to the use of psychotropic medications as these may exacerbate the symptoms. Never use medication without the advice and supervision of a licensed physician.

Devotional

When you are afraid of the person who once would have never threatened or hurt you, it is a devastating and lonesome experience. You know that if he were thinking clearly he would not think of harming you. You want to do the right thing, but how do you know what to do?

When you face difficult decisions, remember God's promise: "If any of you lacks wisdom, he should ask God, who gives generously to all without finding fault, and it will be given to him" (James 1:5).

God has promised to give us guidance in our decision-making. That doesn't mean we pray and then wait for God to telephone us with the answer. But when we sincerely pray for wisdom, then study God's Word and ask the advice of Christian friends, slowly God reveals the right path to us.

Proverbs 3:5-6 also contains a great promise to remember: "Trust in the Lord with all your heart and lean not on your own understanding; in all your ways acknowledge Him, and He will make your paths straight."

HALLUCINATION

I came to the realization that Mary needed medical attention when I observed her conversing with someone in the room who obviously wasn't there. She looked at me as if in disbelief, puzzled that I was unable to clearly see who she was conversing with in the corner. These imaginary people seem to be popping in more often. At first, I thought maybe I was crazy.

Practical Suggestions

Hallucinations are sensory perceptions for which there is no external stimulus. Caregivers should reinforce reality by focusing on the here-and-now and attempting to intervene with the hallucinating person by redirecting his or her attention. Attempt to refocus the direction from the delusional thought process to a real situation.

Be aware of the individual's personal space needs, and avoid making him or her feel threatened or trapped. Reality orientation techniques may be useful, reinforcing the who, what, and where of the situation. Avoid disagreeing with the individual, as arguing will only make matters worse. Medical attention may be necessary if the hallucinations continue.

Devotional

While you do your best to bring the one for whom you are caring back to reality, remember that there is an unseen spiritual world. The Bible urges us to focus "not on what is seen, but on what is unseen. For what is seen is temporary, but what is unseen is eternal" (II Corinthians 4:18).

Lee Carter Maynard, a godly evangelist, lay dying at the age of 94. His secretary sat beside his bed comforting him. Just before he breathed his last, Brother Maynard brightened, and with a burst of energy said. "I see it! It's beautiful! Do you see it?" Then he died. Those closest to Lee Carter Maynard were confident that he was given a glimpse of heaven just before he died.

When your loved one experiences hallucinations, he or she needs to be tactfully brought back to reality. But use that experience to remind yourself there is a spirit world that is real. This physical world will one day pass away, so it is the wise person who sets his mind "on things above, not on earthly things" (Colossians 3:2).

INTIMACY

In the support group last week, we were all asked what it was about this disease that affected us most as caregivers. I sat there for a moment and realized that I miss the personal, intimate relationship that I had with my husband. He no longer puts his arms around me or hugs me as he used to do. When I try to hold his hand, I feel his uneasiness.

Practical Suggestions

Alzheimer's Disease gradually robs the individual of his or her personality. As the disease progresses, the person may experience a decreased ability to be intimate with his or her spouse. The caregiver may go through emotional periods of emptiness where his or her personal needs are not met.

A spouse's needs for intimacy and sexual fulfillment usually result in frustration. Caregivers may feel trapped and often tend to become isolated. This isolation may develop as a result of the impaired individual's growing dependence on the caregiver and a higher risk of embarrassing behaviors.

Caregivers should understand the effects that this disease has on the patient's personality. These changes, if not recognized and addressed, may pose significant problems for their relationship.

Devotional

It is possible to be lonely in a crowd. My loneliest experience came when I first went to college. I had never been away from home for more than five days. Suddenly I was 350 miles from home, separated from my parents, my family and my girlfriend with no chance to go home for nearly three weeks. There were plenty of other people there at college — in fact, I had two roommates. But no one knew me or really cared about me. I can remember turning the radio to KDKA in Pittsburgh and straining to hear through the static the familiar sounds of a Pittsburgh Pirates baseball game. At other times, I would lie in the darkness and wipe away a tear. I learned that you can be surrounded by people and still be lonely.

You might be physically close to your mate, but if his or her personality has changed, you can experience an extreme loneliness that few people could understand.

At those times of loneliness, remember God's promises:

"A man of many companions may come to ruin, but there is a friend who sticks closer than a brother" (Proverbs 18:24).

God said, "Never will I leave you, never will I forsake you" (Hebrews 13:5).

Jesus promised, "Come to me, all you who are weary and burdened, and I will give you rest. Take my yoke upon you and learn from me, for I am gentle and humble in heart, and you will find rest for your souls" (Matthew 11:28-29).

A missionary to the Kiamichi Indians in Oklahoma told about stopping to see an old Indian squaw who had become a Christian. She was sitting alone on the front porch of the cabin when the missionary arrived. When he got out of his car he called out to her, "Are you alone?"

She responded, "Just me and Jesus, son. Just me and Jesus."

What a friend we have in Jesus,

All our sins and griefs to bear.

What a privilege to carry

Everything to God in prayer.

PLACEMENT

My overall goal for caring for Jim was to keep him out of a nursing home at whatever cost. I'd heard so many horror stories about the experiences of others that I really didn't want any part of them. How was I to know that Jim would begin to develop bedsores. His physical condition was more than I could handle. I feel guilty knowing that I can no longer care for him at home.

Practical Suggestions

The consideration of nursing home placement is without a doubt one of the most difficult decisions facing caregivers and their families. In many situations, caregivers have risked their own emotional and physical well-being attempting to keep their loved ones at home.

More often than not it is a major crisis, rather than planning, that prompts the caregiver into making this decision. Personal attitudes regarding nursing homes seem to have some overall effect on the outcome of the experience.

The individual is likely to adjust better to the placement if it occurs when the person is still able to adjust and cope with the new surroundings. Caregivers should explore and evaluate appropriate facilities to see which will best serve their needs and the patient's.

When looking for a nursing home, ask the administrator or staff to show you a copy of their latest state survey report. This document can provide you with valuable information regarding the facility's past operational and patient care performance. Another good source of input about the facility can come from discussions and personal experiences with other residents and their families.

Devotional

When my son was four years old, he had to have corrective eye surgery. He was old enough to understand it was for his benefit. When the doctor came to the room to take him to surgery, my son grabbed me around the neck and said, "Daddy, I love you. Please don't let them take me away." I couldn't get him to understand it was for his own good. It was hard to let him go, but I did because I cared for him.

It is a difficult experience for a caregiver to release a loved one to a nursing home. It is heartbreaking to walk away when the one you love so much feels confused or let down. But often you have decided to do the most loving thing. You are acknowledging your own limitations in a situation that you cannot control and providing the best care you can for your loved one.

When Jesus was leaving this earth, he assured us that the Holy Spirit would be with us to be a comforter. And He promised that He would some day return to take us with Him to the Father's house, where we will be reunited with those we love for eternity (John 14).

FABRICATION

I listened to my wife the other day as she explained to our neighbors where we had been on vacation. I was amazed at how she made up things as she spoke. The details of our trip were so fabricated. If you hadn't known better, you'd think we really did do all of those things.

Practical Suggestions

As this disease progresses, the individual may find it difficult to accurately articulate what he or she is trying to express. This behavior is not intentional nor malicious, but rather a part of the disease process.

Expressions of thoughts and events are intermingled with fictitious comments as the person has difficulty filling in gaps. Encourage the person to speak slowly and remove any unnecessary background noise. Allow the individual to have plenty of response time before asking the same question.

Paraphasia, where the individual associates the meaning of one word with another, is quite common. Through a process of decoding, the caregiver may be able to break the code of the newly assigned words and better understand the message. Attempt to clarify the facts of the story unless it appears to be upsetting to the person.

Devotional

To lie is to deliberately misrepresent the truth. If I am unaware that my watch is broken and I give someone the incorrect time, I have not lied because I am not deliberately misrepresenting the truth. However, if I know my watch is broken and someone asks what time I arrived home last night, I would be lying to say, "According to my watch it was midnight." Though I may be relating facts that are true, I am deliberately misrepresenting the complete truth.

When someone's mind is not functioning properly, he or she may not relate all the facts accurately, but it is not a deliberate attempt to misrepresent the truth. At the time, it is best for caregiver to show patience and understanding rather than getting angry or embarrassed, or attempting to correct the facts immediately. The Bible says we should "love truth and peace" (Zechariah 8:19).

Remember, though, that while one suffering from Alzheimer's will not be held accountable for his inaccuracies, that does not exempt you from the need to be honest. "Each of you must put off falsehood and speak truthfully to his neighbor, for we are all members of one body" (Ephesians 4:25).

TREMORS

Tom can barely hold the cup in his hands steadily, without spilling his drink everywhere. Sometimes his entire body shakes uncontrollably. I've noticed recently that he's started this tapping motion with his hands and feet. It's almost rhythmic, yet he says he has no control over this behavior.

Practical Suggestions

Tremors and shaking behavior may sometimes be perceived as nervous gestures. There may be a number of different causes for this type of activity. Individuals with Alzheimer's Disease may exhibit Parkinson-type symptoms. This is characterized by the loss of mobility and motor control.

Careful consideration of safety issues should be made, especially when individuals are unsteady on their feet and find it difficult to maneuver. A medical consultation is usually warranted to assess the severity of the problem. Neurological problems may exist which can be compounded through side-effects of certain medications.

Devotional

The apostle Paul wrote, "Now we know that if the earthly tent we live in is destroyed, we have a building from God, an eternal house in heaven, not built by human hands" (II Corinthians 5.1). As our bodies age, it is frustrating that we cannot stop the process. But trembling hands, fading eyesight and slowed reaction times are all reminders that our physical bodies are just tents. Tents are temporary. They're not comfortable. They offer little protection.

When this earthly tent begins to deteriorate we need to rejoice that God promises a new building — a new secure, eternal, comfortable body in which to live in heaven.

Remember the old song, "This Ol' House"? You would sing, "This ol' house is getting kinda weary, this ol' house is getting kinda worn." The song concluded with this: "Ain't gonna need this house no longer, ain't gonna need this house no more . . . I'm getting ready to meet the Lord!"

"Listen, I tell you a mystery: We will not all sleep, but we will all be changed — in a flash, in the twinkling of an eye, at the last trumpet. For the trumpet will sound, the dead will be raised imperishable, and we will be changed. For the perishable must clothe itself with the imperishable, and the mortal with immortality . . . then the saying that is written will come true: 'Death has been swallowed up in victory' " (I Corinthians 15:51-54).

Former President John Adams was asked in his later years how he was doing. He responded, "John Adams is doing fine, thank you. But the house I live in is about to give way." Rejoice today that God promises us new bodies in heaven.

When we've been there ten thousand years,

Bright shining as the sun,

We've no less days to sing God's praise

Than when we first begun.

AGNOSIA
(RECOGNITION)

My wife is gradually losing her ability to recognize that I am her husband. The other day she questioned me as to who the stranger was in our bathroom. She no longer realizes that it was her image she saw in the mirror.

Practical Suggestions

Agnosia is characterized by the lack of sensory and perceptual ability of the individual to recognize objects — including people. The person with Alzheimer's Disease gradually loses his or her ability to recognize familiar faces, including spouses of many years.

It is not uncommon for law enforcement officers to be called to the scene of a possible break in only to find the spouse of many years believed to be the burglar. This behavior can be disheartening for the caregiver who has become physically and emotionally exhausted by caring for this person.

Familiar items and landmarks may be difficult to recognize. Caregivers should calmly attempt to clarify and reinforce those items in question, being careful not to upset the patient. Correct distorted statements with factual comments that accurately identify who the people are and what items the person is discussing.

Devotional

People sometimes ask me if we will recognize each other in heaven. That seems like a silly question because, although I know I will have changed for the better, if you don't recognize me, I'll tell you who I am! I want you to know I'm there!

Paul said, "Now I know in part; then I shall know fully, even as I am fully known" (I Corinthians 13:12). The Bible tells us that we will sit down with Abraham, Isaac and Jacob in the Kingdom. If those men are identifiable, I believe we will recognize each other as well.

Our eternal hope is that one day God will restore our bodies and our mental capacities and we will spend eternity with Him and our loved ones. I was teaching a men's Bible study on the subject of death and dying when I asked the older men present, "Do you fear dying more or less as you get older?" They all agreed that one fears dying less with age. "Why is that?" I asked.

Butch Dabney, a grand Christian of 76 years, said, "It's because you've got more friends in heaven than you've got on earth!"

"Therefore, my dear brothers, stand firm. Let nothing move you. Always give yourselves fully to the work of the Lord, because you know that your labor in the Lord is not in vain" (I Corinthians 15:58).

Alzheimer's Disease Overview

Impact of Alzheimer's Disease

In the past several years a lot of research has taken place in an attempt to uncover the cause and to find a possible cure for Alzheimer's disease. Though we've made major strides in the research arena, there is still a lot that we don't know about this deadly illness. We do know that Alzheimer's disease is a progressive brain disorder that was first described in 1907 by Aloise Alzheimer, a German neurologist. Its primary symptom and hallmark characteristic is memory impairment. Without a known cure, this disease affects over 4 million American adults and is the fourth leading cause of adult death in this country. Approximately 100,000 lives are taken each year by this devastating illness. Some health experts predict that by the year 2040, an estimated 12 to 14 million people have Alzheimer's disease. Over half of the current nursing home residents in this country are also believed to be suffering from Alzheimer's disease. With the increased aging of our society it's a sure fact that this percentage will continue to grow in the future.

Disease Overview

It is important to note that Alzheimer's disease is not just an occasional forgetfulness, but rather an ongoing impairment with one's memory. Over a period of time this disease renders the individual unable to take care of personal needs essential for daily functioning and survival. *My husband is a skeletal reminder of a person who once was,* is the way one caregiver described the effects of this disease on her spouse. How tragic, to witness the sometimes slow deterioration of a person who once was so full of vigor and life. Worse yet, is to observe the sometimes devastating effects that this disease has on the caregiver. It's no wonder that this disease is said to have two victims, the individual afflicted and the caregiver.

Early Warning Signals

Individuals afflicted with this disease are often very much aware in the early stages that something just isn't right. They just can't quite figure it out. Family members are likely to pass off the slowed speech or the miscalculated accounting of events to a "normal" aging process or to the need for the individual to have more rest. The signs and symptoms that the individual is exhibiting are not normal aging behaviors; rather, they are a direct result of a disease process. Compounding the problem of diagnosis is the keen ability of the individual to cover up his or her impairments. Unfortunately, this allows the disease to run it's course without medical or family intervention. Early warning signals of this disease include an increased tendency to misplace things. Confusion and the inability to stay on task are also common symptoms. The individual may also begin to have difficulty in expressing himself and may appear to be at a loss with putting complete sentences together. Over a period of time, familiar landmarks in their neighborhood, even their own home, may be forgotten and may pose serious safety concerns.

Stages of Alzheimer's Disease

Stage One

Alzheimer's disease is clinically categorized into three stages, early or stage one, middle or stage two, and late or stage three. Symptoms of the these stages may often be inter-changeable; however, there is usually a marked deterioration in the individual's functioning level from one stage to the next. Plateaus or periods where the individual's condition does not appear to worsen or may even appear to slightly improve may be common. This roller-coaster type of behavior often gives a false sense of hope to the afflicted individual and to his or her family members. Symptoms of stage one include memory loss, especially with recent events rather than events that took place years ago. Information and specific details from years gone by may be easily recalled; however, the individual may have diffi-culty remembering details about an event that just recently occurred. The person with Alzheimer's disease may also have difficulty with orientation to time and can exhibit poor judgment in making decisions. One's use of language as it relates to expressing and articulating a particular message may become impaired. The person may also have difficulty putting together complete sentences. During this stage the person with Alzheimer's disease may become careless in their actions and physical appearance. Reduced attention to personal dress and hygiene becomes noticeable to others. As the disease progresses the individual begins to have more difficulty staying on task, remembering and acting responsibly. Caregivers are also faced with the increased responsibility of making critical decisions that the individual is no longer able to make on their own.

Stage Two

It is usually during the latter part of stage one or the early part of stage two that a major crisis occurs. This ususally occurs in the form of a behavioral outburst that presents itself as a major dilemna for the caregiver, such as a physical confrontation, a wandering episode or some other type of inappropriate activity. Odd or peculiar behaviors become more noticeable due to the persons inability to cover up his or her personal mistakes. It is usually at this time that the individual is persuaded to seek medical attention. Unfortunately, this is not always an easy task for the caregiver nor freely accepted by the individual afflicted. This can often be an experience met with much resistance directed towards the caregiver. During this stage the person gradually becomes more disoriented and confused. Restless behavior at night as well as reversed sleep patterns can pose a tremendous challenge to the caregiver and their family. It is also during this stage that the individual has difficulty with communication, both sending as well as receiving messages. Caregivers must enhance their skills to better anticipate and perceive the specific needs of the patient. Specific interventions that may work for the caregiver one day may be totally ineffective the next. As the disease progresses, social behaviors such as proper dress and toileting may become forgotten. When this occurs, it can present embarrassing moments for the person and for his or her family. Disrobing in public often presents additional stress and strain on the caregiver and their family members. Poor judgment and the inability to stay on task also increases the likelihood of an accident and may pose serious safety concerns for the person with Alzheimer's. Episodes of wandering behavior pose one of the most significant safety concerns since the person is no longer able to assess and evaluate the risks of danger in their surroundings. Unfortunately, a number of fatalities are recorded each year as a direct result of a wandering episode.

Stage Three

During stage three, or the final stage of Alzheimer's disease, the individual has now become totally dependent on others for complete care. The person is now unable to communicate with others, and long-standing acquaintances, even one's spouse of many years, are now total strangers. There is a marked deterioration in the individual's appearance with considerable weight loss and lack of control with both bowel and bladder functioning. Ultimately the person becomes totally helpless and bedridden, with pneumonia likely being the cause of death due to poor circulation. By now the span of time for the three stages of this disease may have been from two to twenty years.

Caregiver Attributes

Though personal experiences have shown that no two people diagnosed with this disease will be exactly alike, there are some common attributes of caregivers that stand out. One's personal faith and a strong spiritual support system appear to more effectively allow the caregiver to deal with the difficult role of caregiving. Other elements of caregiving that reduce the risk of burnout include the need to excel in the following areas:

Assessment
Security
Stimulation
Patience
Anticipation
Communication
Perception